SlimCalmSexy
YOGA

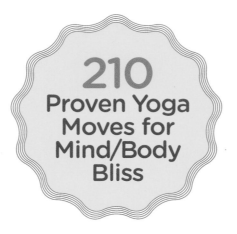

210
Proven Yoga Moves for Mind/Body Bliss

By TARA STILES

RODALE®

Rodale books may be purchased for business or promotional use or for special sales. For information, please write to:
Special Markets Department, Rodale Inc., 733 Third Avenue, New York, NY 10017

Women's Health is a registered trademark of Rodale Inc.

Printed in the United States of America
Rodale Inc. makes every effort to use acid-free ⊗, recycled paper ♻.

**Book design by Mike Smith,
with George Karabotsos, design director of Men's Health and Women's Health Books**

Photographs by Beth Bischoff

Library of Congress Cataloging-in-Publication Data

Stiles, Tara.
    Slim calm sexy yoga : 210 Proven Yoga Moves for Mind/Body Bliss / Tara Stiles.
        p.   cm.
    Includes index.
    ISBN-13: 978-1-60529-556-5   paperback
    ISBN-10: 1-60529-556-6   paperback
    1. Yoga. I. Title.
    RA781.7.S75   2010
    613.7—dc22

Distributed to the trade by Macmillan

    4 6 8 10 9 7 5 3   paperback

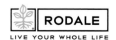

LIVE YOUR WHOLE LIFE

We inspire and enable people to improve their lives and the world around them.
For more of our products visit **rodalebooks.com**

For Grandma Gray and
Grandma Richardson, who
inspire my practice every day.

And for Molly and Abby,
who I hope my practice
will inspire one day.

Acknowledgments

I'm grateful to countless individuals who have inspired and led me to the place in my life that made this book possible. Everyone who has encouraged, discouraged, or otherwise nudged me along the way has shaped my ability to communicate and authenticate the practice of yoga and conscious living.

Thanks for the focused effort and guidance of Leah Flickinger, editor extraordinaire. Thanks to Michele Promaulayko, Steve Perrine, Dave Zinczenko, Debbie McHugh, Beth Bischoff, George Karabotsos, Mike Smith, Thea Palad, Michiko Boorberg (cuz), Lauren Saldutti, Beth Bazar, Erana Bumbardatore, Sarah Rozen, Erin Williams, Chris Krogermeier, Brooke Myers, Sara Cox, Jayme Lynes, Jay Ehrlich, Julie Stewart, and Jen Ator. Without this talented group, this book would not exist.

Thanks to Liezl Panlilio, Namrata Tripathi, Verena Von Pfetten, Lindsay Mannering, Fernanda Hess, Tiffany West, Galiya Khabibullina, and Kate Creeden Neckel for the inspiration, time, energy, and story-sharing that brought this project to life. Thanks to everyone who practices yoga at Strala, or with me via podcast or other means. I am able to do what I do because of your support and encouragement.

Thanks to Ms. Zima, whose graceful awareness inspired me to be my best. Thanks to Rory Foster for noticing my bend toward yoga and guiding me into further studies. Thanks to Jane Fonda for being awesome. Thanks to Piper Kerman and Larry Smith for finding me again. Thanks to Ed and Deb Shapiro, my spiritual godparents. Thanks to Deepak Chopra for your friendship and partnership that keeps reminding me to have confidence in myself. Thanks to Will Hobbs for believing in me and for all your hard work to convince others to do the same. Thanks to Mom, Dad, Chad, and the rest of the family for putting up with me from day one and instilling the common sense I take for granted. Special thanks to Kristin Dollard for pulling me into Rodale as an aspiring ex-model/dancer-turned-blogger.

And thanks, Michael, for always being there.

Contents

Slim. Calm. Sexy.
Wouldn't it be fantastic to feel that way all the time?

The reality is that we're often too busy, too tired, too stressed to do what it takes to get those results. Things like eating well, exercising, even just taking a deep breath now and then seem beyond our grasp in the hectic world we live in. And that hectic way of living leads to an endless cycle of stress, exhaustion, weight gain, anxiety, and frustration. There goes slim, calm, sexy.

Well, go ahead and take that nice long, deep breath.

Because I've got some great news: There is something you can do to radiate slim, calm, sexy from the inside out—in just 15 minutes a day. It's a revolutionary new approach to the ancient discipline of yoga, and it's proven by research to work.

With this simple guide, I'll teach you how to focus on the little things that make your life seem hard—a sore back, a pounding head, a growling stomach, even a nagging boss—and show you how to turn them around in just 15 minutes a day. My approach is based on harnessing the healing power of yoga and applying it in the most targeted way possible—fixing whatever hurts you, stresses you, or makes you sad, in less time than it takes to wash and dry your hair.

And you will be amazed at how it will transform you.

There's a reason I believe in the 15-minute yoga fix. See, I know exactly what it's like to think you're too stressed, too busy, and too exhausted to feel slim, calm, or anywhere close to sexy. So before I get into the details of how yoga will change your life, let me tell you a little something about how it changed mine.

I grew up in rural Illinois, and there weren't many kids to hang out with, so I spent a lot of time on my own scrambling up trees, sitting, thinking, and just breathing as I soaked in the nature that surrounded me. I honestly believe that all that time I spent alone in the treetops contemplating the mysteries of the universe was my first experience with what I now know as meditation. But it wasn't until I was in my teens and enrolled in a rigorous classical dance program that I had formal contact with yoga. Once a week, as part of our training, a yoga teacher sat serenely in front of the group leading us through poses and meditations to relax our tightly wound bodies. And while I loved to dance, doing yoga made me feel more alive than endless pliés at the barre. It was like being back up in the trees. I felt at home.

My story would be nice and simple if I could tell you that once I discovered yoga, I'd found my calling and lived happily ever after. But in real life, signs are not always so clear, and the paths we start on aren't always so easy to jump off.

I had chosen classical dance as my path at an early age. Like a lot of little girls, I wanted to be a ballerina almost as soon as I could walk. I was a born performer with natural grace and skill, gifts that served me well in my small-town recitals. It was a good fit—until I saw how competitive the real world of dance is.

I started formal training at a professional level when I was 10, and I found myself surrounded by ballerinas who had trained in far more hard-core programs than I had. To keep up, I had to work doubly hard. And it was tough not to compare myself obsessively with these girls. My confidence shriveled. By the time I was in my late teens, I'd evolved from a happy, intuitive kid into an insecure, people-pleasing young adult.

It didn't help that at 5 feet 9 inches tall, I was considered a giant in the world of ballet. In pointe shoes, I towered over all my potential dance partners. (Yes, dancer guys are on the small side.) In a roomful of petite girls, I felt like a big, clumsy monster. I grew to dislike my body and began to have doubts about my talent and purpose. My self-esteem plummeted.

At least my height served one purpose: Onstage I was hard to miss. A Chicago photographer took notice, and we did a fashion-inspired ballet shoot. He showed the pictures to an agent, and I signed with Aria models (now the prestigious Ford agency) and started to work in magazines and TV commercials. But when I quit dance and moved to New York City in the summer of 2000 (I was 20) to model full-time, things on the confidence front didn't get much better.

Don't get me wrong. Many people would consider a modeling contract in New York a dream come true. And it was definitely an exciting time, full of glitz and glam. But as yoga took a backseat to endless go-sees and photo shoots, I continued to struggle with my self-worth and started to feel lost. I was 800 miles from my family and trying to survive in a Chutes and Ladders industry. My job description was to be slim, calm, and sexy, but let me tell you, often I felt nothing like that. I felt misplaced, misunderstood, and unfulfilled.

Then one day, a couple of years after moving to New York City, I had a moment of clarity. I was doing insanely long back-to-back shoots (a music video shoot all night, straight to a Lady Foot Locker campaign in the morning). I was exhausted to the point of tears. I couldn't and didn't want to continue down the path I was on. It had no substantial meaning for me and didn't fuel me with anything positive. I had seen much more exciting things meditating in the trees and on the mat in yoga class. I began to wonder if yoga could bring me back to myself.

It didn't happen overnight, but soon after I made yoga a priority in my life, I started feeling alive again. The physicality of yoga reminded me how to feel good in my body. Its meditative side made me feel good in my head. Practicing yoga helped me figure out how to sync up my body and mind so I could return to my own intuitive sense of well-being, the one I'd had so naturally as a kid. I'd forgotten what I was capable of, but once I was back to a regular practice, I realized I was finally on the right path to a healthy and satisfying life. It was a game changer.

In the past decade, I've made up for lost time. I've devoured the teachings of such major players as Paramahansa Yogananda, Krishna Das, Ram Dass, Dharma Mittra, and many other meditation masters, mystics, and healers. I continue to explore, meditate, and learn through my own practices and the wisdom of others. I still model now and then, but I've devoted my life to helping other people through yoga. Today I run my own studio, called Strala Yoga, in New York City, where I teach some of the most successful, hard-charging people in the world—from busy executives to professional actors to members of the military—to be slim, calm, and sexy.

And I want to teach you, too.

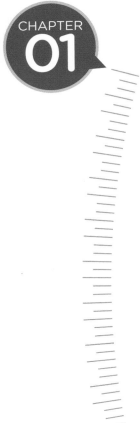

15 minutes to a slimmer, calmer, sexier you!

Your transformation starts here

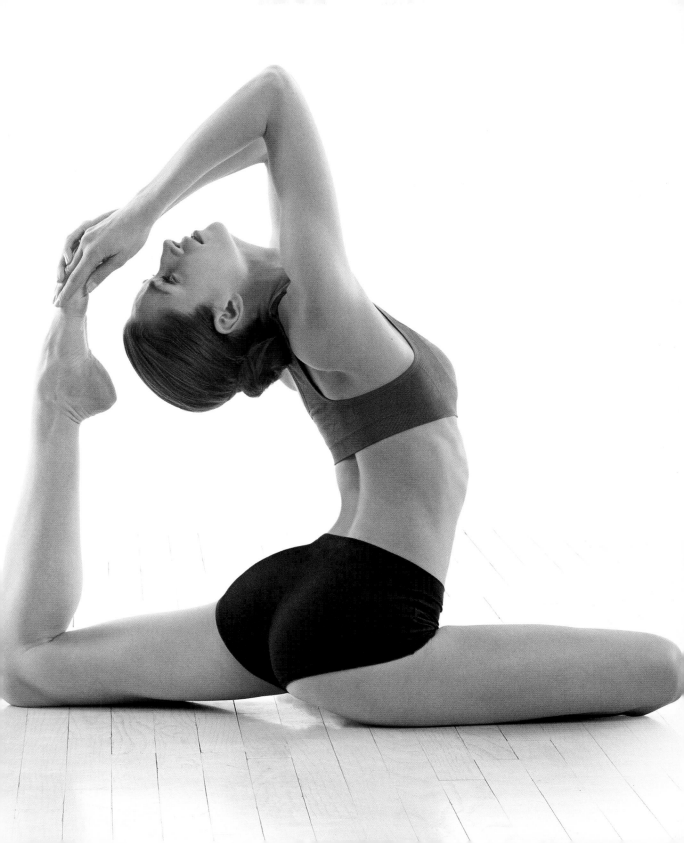

Here's my promise: If you let it, yoga can change your life. Maybe you've always thought yoga is reserved only for the superskinny, or for Hindu converts who make regular pilgrimages to India. Maybe you think it's just a bunch of stretching and deep breathing, and a total nonworkout.

But before you dismiss it, consider this: Yoga's many benefits—including a slimmer body, stronger immunity, lower blood pressure, improved mood, better sex, and more—are backed by a growing pile of research. There are very real and exciting results.

If you're already a yoga regular, no doubt you're familiar with that amazing feeling you get right after a class. Some people call it the yoga buzz. And scientists have discovered the potent mechanism behind it: Turns out, yoga has a direct effect on your brain. It actually raises levels of a chemical in your noggin called gamma-aminobutyric acid (GABA), which is linked to well-being. Researchers at Boston University School of Medicine and McLean Hospital used MRI scans to measure baseline GABA levels in study volunteers. The scientists then asked half of them to do an hour of yoga while the others read a book. When the participants were rescanned afterward, the yogis had increased their GABA levels by an average of 27 percent, whereas the bookworms showed no change. Those are some serious feel-good results.

In another study, UCLA researchers measured significant and immediate mood changes in people who had just taken a yoga class. Their bad moods decreased while their good moods increased, and they were less tired and more energetic. That's good stuff. It happens each time you practice, and you can be practicing all the time, whether you are on your yoga mat or not.

I'll share more results like this throughout the book, though once you get into a full-on yoga kick, you may not feel the need to have doctors and studies tell you what's good for you. You'll feel the difference yourself. Yoga has a way of waking up your intuition about your own health and well-being. But, for the science-minded among you, consider these compelling facts.

Yoga Will Make You Slimmer

There is a common misunderstanding that yoga isn't effective for weight loss. I am here to tell you that that couldn't be further from the truth. For starters, you will sweat, blast calories, and tone and shape your entire body, especially if you practice a more physically active style of yoga, such as ashtanga, Vinyasa, or Bikram (hot yoga). In fact, you'll burn 400 calories in a 90-minute Bikram class, roughly the same as in 40 minutes of running at a moderate pace—but with a lot less stress on your body.

That said, calorie burning is not where the bulk of yoga's weight-loss power lies. An added benefit, even from practicing more gentle styles of yoga and meditation, is that it helps you get a handle on what your body needs to be healthy and feel good.

OK, I don't blame you if you're thinking, "That sounds like bullsh--. What if my body *needs* french fries?" I totally get that. But believe me when I tell you that doing yoga gives you a special fat-fighting power. Here's how it works: Yoga requires your full attention and concentration to move through the poses and to hold them. (Just try staying in plank pose while obsessing over those boots you saw at Anthropologie.) Cultivating attention and awareness on the yoga mat shines a spotlight on habits and behaviors off the mat, including choices about what—and how much—is for dinner. And over time, a regular yoga practice will sharpen your ability to gauge how hungry or full you are. (Do

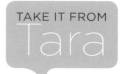

TAKE IT FROM
Tara

GUIDING BREATH

The practice of yoga brings you back to YOU, where all the good stuff is. When you rest your attention on your breath, instead of your thinking, your creativity and intuition have room to surface.

Try it now. Close your eyes and follow your breath for a moment and see where it leads you. When you follow your breath, your instincts kick in and help guide you to the things you need to stay healthy.

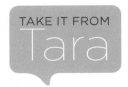

TAKE IT FROM
Tara

TRY IT, YOU'LL LIKE IT

Yoga is experiental. No matter how much I can try to persuade you that it works, you have to try it yourself and see what happens. The good news is that, each time you practice, you'll feel less stressed and more energized.

you really need that piece of chocolate lava cake?)

Still skeptical? Maybe this will help. A recent study published in the *Journal of the American Dietetic Association* found a strong association between yoga practice and weight control, and researchers attribute it simply to eating "mindfully." Down dog devotees, they say, learn to stay calm in the face of discomfort, and that tendency spills over into other parts of their lives—making it easier to turn down that cake (or fries), no matter how good it looks.

What's more, the study found no such link between mindful eating and other types of physical activity, such as walking or running. I can vouch for this from personal experience. When I first moved to New York City from Chicago, I went through a brief gym phase, alternating gym workouts with occasional yoga. After a while I started noticing an interesting pattern. When I finished a session on the elliptical, I'd grab takeout or a quick sandwich from a deli. I wouldn't think much about what I was eating or why. I was hungry, it was convenient, decision made.

But after yoga class, my behavior was different. I'd find myself gravitating toward fruit or shopping for organic greens so I could make a salad creation at home. I was hyperaware of how my body and mind felt after

yoga—cleansed and healthy—and wanted to keep them that way.

There's nothing mystical going on here. Practicing mindless activity leads to mindless behavior—yes, even eating. Most cardio exercise, particularly the kind you do on gym equipment, quickly becomes rote, making it super-easy for you to zone out completely and not think about how you make decisions. On the other hand, practicing a mindful activity (like yoga) leads to consciously choosing behaviors that make your body feel good.

Another crucial factor in yoga's pound-crushing power is that it's proven to reduce the one thing that 43 percent of Americans say makes them overeat. That one thing? Stress.

I'll get into the fascinating stress-food-weight connection in much greater detail in Chapter 4, but rest assured that there's plenty of evidence to support the idea that practicing yoga will slim you down by settling you down.

Which leads me to . . .

Yoga Will Make You Calmer

Every day, people walk into the yoga studio all bottled up with stress. Every day, they walk out happy and calm. Stress will always be a part of life. There's no way to make it disappear completely. (I wish!) But yoga is proven to help you handle it better. In a 2009 study published in the journal *Health Education and Behavior*, office workers who took part in a 6-week yoga and meditation program reported significantly lower stress levels and improved sleep quality. Sitting up and paying attention to your breath for 5 minutes before bedtime leads to a more restful sleep than watching reruns of *Frasier* until your eyes can't stay open. Likewise, 5 minutes of yoga when you wake up, before you start checking your e-mail and making breakfast, sets your mind in a calm state for the day.

And the more yoga you practice, the better your body will handle stress, which has major implications for your overall health. A ground-breaking study published in 2010 by Ohio State University scientists looked at yoga's role in reducing inflammation. (Inflammation signals several serious health conditions, including diabetes, heart disease, and osteoporosis, and is strongly influenced by stress.) Study participants were divided into two groups: yoga practitioners with at least 2 years of experience and yoga novices. Scientists gauged inflammation by measuring blood levels of several chemicals, including one called interleukin-6 (IL-6), high levels of which have been linked to chronic stress. The novices' IL-6 levels at the beginning of the study were 41 percent higher than those of the expert yogis. What's more, when exposed to stressful situations like immersing their feet in freezing water or solving difficult math equations, the novices produced nearly 25 percent more IL-6 than the yoga experts did. The researchers aren't sure what aspect of practicing yoga confers the benefit but suggest that yoga is a powerful stress buster that will lead to a longer, healthier life.

If work, family, or problems with a friend or partner are the cause of your stress, yoga can help you paint a clearer picture of what is actually going on and guide you to your best path. Yoga teaches you how to focus and pay attention to detail. You have to learn to stack your arms, legs, spine, and neck in correct alignment so you can stay balanced. You also have to maintain your attention and make adjustments so you don't fall over. It forces you to focus on how your body and mind feel, along with how to make adjustments that optimize that feeling. This translates directly into your life off the mat. It helps you see what's in front of you more clearly so you can act from a grounded place and make good decisions. This is called mindfulness, and you'll hear a lot more about it later in the book. It comes into play every time you practice yoga, and it's a very good thing.

Yoga Will Make You Feel Sexier

Seeing a slimmer, calmer you gazing out from the mirror goes a long way toward upping your confidence and making you feel beautiful. But yoga's sexy side effects are about much more than through-the-roof confidence and glowing skin (though your skin really will start to glow; I'll share the proof in Chapter 8).

Yoga not only makes you feel like a vixen, it also physically changes your body from the inside out so that you experience pleasure in a whole new way. Whether you're into bedroom gymnastics or more traditional lovemaking, all the added strength, flexibility, and endurance you gain with yoga practice will lead to amazing times between the sheets. And if you're lucky enough to have a partner who practices yoga with you, you might want to brace yourself for the orgasm jackpot. Need a better reason to drag your date to yoga? (Be careful, you might not make it to dinner.)

True story: I met my husband at yoga camp in a retreat center a train ride away from New York City. It was a weekend of positive yoga energy. One of my all-time favorite people, Krishna Das (I call him the rock star of yoga), spoke and sang. And one of the masters I most admire, Dharma Mittra, who has been teaching in New York City since the 1970s, was leading classes.

There I was in my sweatpants, no makeup, soaking up the atmosphere, totally on vacation from my mind, when I spotted Mike from across the room. It's not often you find a hot and "normal-looking" dude at a yoga retreat, but the last thing I was interested in that weekend was meeting someone.

All the eye contact started getting awkward, and then I noticed that we had something in common: chocolate. I'd snuck some M&Ms into camp knowing there wouldn't be much dessert available, and wouldn't you know it, he was furtively making his way through a stash of Easter chocolate he'd brought to a Krishna Das talk. My stash was running low. Conversation starter taken care of.

When you stop looking and quiet your mind, intuition and awareness take hold, and good stuff happens. It's the same with love. I blush easily when I talk about sex, especially my own sex life, but I will divulge that it is a very good idea to find a partner who practices a lot of yoga.

You don't have to go to yoga camp (or be a committed Tantra practitioner) to enjoy the sexy side effects of yoga. All that time on the mat spent cultivating focus, looking inward, and moving and breathing deeply leads to beaming confidence and sensuality, whether you're walking down the street or getting your groove on in the bedroom. A 2009 study published in the *Journal of Sexual Medicine* found that women who followed a 12-week yoga program reported significant improvements in desire, arousal, lubrication, sexual satisfaction, and orgasm.

Yoga's influence on your orgasms is twofold. In strengthening your core, you gain greater control over your pelvic floor muscles and sex organs. Harnessing this during sex helps you climax more magnificently. Regular yoga practice also reduces muscle tension, which, in turn, makes your body more receptive to pleasure.

What You Will Get from This Book

If you are already a yoga convert, you know from direct experience how amazing the benefits of regular practice are. No matter what result you're after—weight loss, less stress, better sex—in *Slim Calm Sexy Yoga* you'll find a targeted program to get it. Best of all, most take just 15 minutes (totally excuse-proof!).

But yoga's many benefits don't end with weight loss, stress reduction, and better sex. A regular yoga practice can have a powerful impact on your health—from curing headaches to easing hangovers to

preventing heart disease. And if you simply want to dazzle the world, you'll find 15-minute yoga fixes that will tone your body or give you smooth, beautiful skin.

Doing the routines in this book is like hitting the reset button on your body and mind any time you need to. By focusing and breathing, you can cultivate awareness and attention, and direct your energy toward your goals. Practicing this way reveals your unique qualities, and part of that yoga buzz everyone raves about is realizing how much potential and power you have. You have the power to live a happy and fulfilled life. You just need to practice—and keep practicing.

I crafted these routines specifically to fit easily into your life. Work at your own pace and around your busy schedule. Five minutes here and 15 minutes there will make a huge difference from your very first deep breath. Just ask some of the clients I've worked with. I'm inspired every day by people who've wholeheartedly embraced a yoga lifestyle—and how it's changed them for the better. On the following pages, I'll introduce you to six real women (a lot like you!) who embody *Slim Calm Sexy Yoga*. You'll see firsthand how a regular yoga practice can do the same for you.

Ready to get started?

CHAPTER 02

bring on the yoga buzz

Three yoga principles
that will change your life—
and how to use them

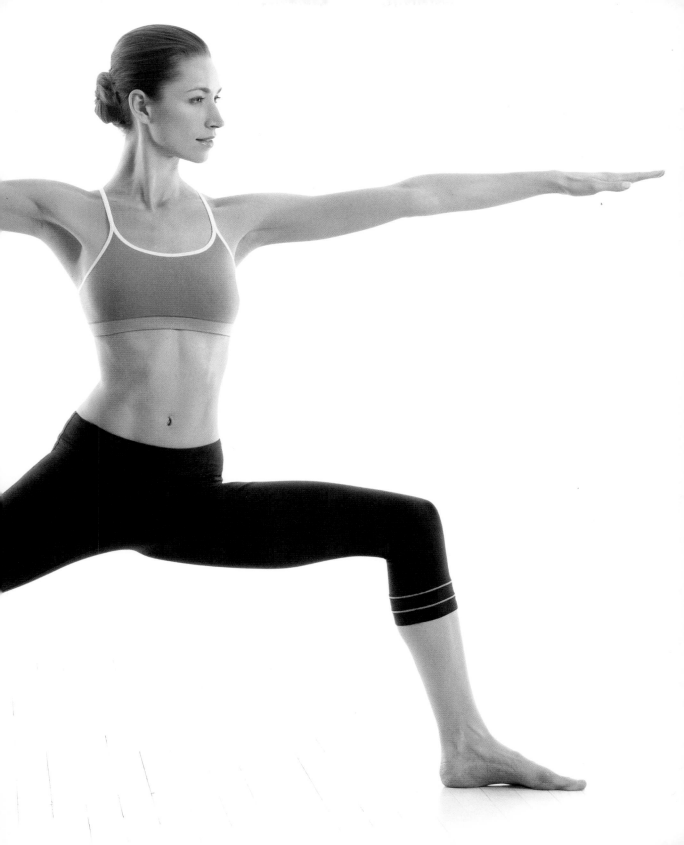

Want to start feeling better than ever?

Want to check your stress at the door, fit into your skinny jeans, do a double take when you catch your reflection in a shop window? Good, because I want to help you get there. But before we delve into the fabulous ways yoga can help you embody *Slim Calm Sexy Yoga*, I want to introduce you to a few principles of yoga that will make your practice a hundred times more effective: breathing, meditation, and alignment.

just **breathe!**

Yoga won't do you much good if you hold your breath through each pose. Your breath has a direct influence on your nervous system. The ancient yogis figured out how to harness it for maximum chill-out effect, and now modern science confirms it: Controlled breathing confers a host of health benefits, including lowering blood pressure, reducing panic attacks, and even minimizing asthma, according to studies presented at an American Psychosomatic Society conference. Slow, deep breathing can restore balance in your nervous system, which is impaired by a number of cardiovascular diseases and stress-related problems.

How does the simple intake of air impart all these benefits? Harvard University's Herbert Benson, MD, one of the first physicians to bring Eastern healing into Western medicine, has shown in his research on high blood pressure that harmful physiological effects can be alleviated by breathing deeply while focusing your mind on a repetitive sound, word, phrase, or movement. Benson dubbed this the relaxation response: a state of deep rest that changes your physical and emotional reaction to stress in a way that can improve health.

If your breathing becomes short and fast during a challenging pose, try to guide it back to long and deep. Your body and mind work best with a steady and deep flow of oxygen. As with yoga, the effects of deep breathing spill over into everyday life. When you're in a tense situation, such as a confrontation with a coworker, what's your natural reaction? If you tend to hold your breath and tense up, you're like most of us. But if you can train yourself to breathe deeply through stressful moments, you will be much more prepared to think and act clearly than if you ball up until the tough situation passes. Deep breathing allows you to stay focused on what's in front of you and deal with it in the most capable way possible. On the flip side, this practice lets you experience good things when they come your way, too.

THE NOSE KNOWS

Breathing for yoga practice is done primarily through the nose. Why? For starters, the nose screens out dust and dirt particles that the mouth can't. Just as you use a filter for drinking water, your nose is your very own natural air filter. Breathing through your nose also controls the amount of air you inhale and exhale. It leads to longer, deeper breathing, which helps you focus more than if you gulp air through your mouth.

Breathing techniques guide and control the amount of air that circulates through your system, which helps to quiet your mind and leaves your body feeling calm and at ease.

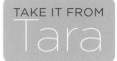
 Sage Secrets | LIFE AND BREATH

ANCIENT YOGA PHILOSOPHY says that you are allotted a certain number of breaths in your life. You can lengthen or shorten your life by how you take those breaths.

Short and fast breathing is the result of living a stressful, out-of-balance existence. This leads to disease and a shortened life. Long, deep breathing keeps your body and mind vibrant and healthy, and allows you to live a long, full life.

Interestingly, animals that breathe slowly, such as the elephant, live for a very long time (up to 80 years, in the pachyderm's case). Ganesha, a Hindu deity prevalent in statue form in many yoga studios, is the lord of success and destroyer of evils and obstacles. Ganesha has an elephant's head, trunk, and ears, and a huge, humanlike potbelly full of breath. He is also worshipped as the god of education, knowledge, wisdom, and wealth.

Deep Breathing

This basic technique will teach you how to take long, deep breaths through the nose. If you are brand new to yoga, you might want to start moving through the poses and meditations in this book using this breathing technique before moving on to ones that are more complex.

the ROUTINE

You can practice deep breathing anytime, including while you are practicing yoga.

Lie flat on your back in corpse pose: legs straight on the floor in front of you, arms relaxed on the mat by your sides. Take a deep breath. /// Exhale all the air out. Pull your lower belly in and hold the air out for a moment. /// Inhale from your lower belly, then up through your middle chest, then your upper chest. Hold all the air in for a moment. /// Slowly exhale, starting with your upper chest, then your middle chest, and finally your belly. Exhale fully, pull your belly in, and hold the air out for a moment. Repeat for a total of 10 breaths.

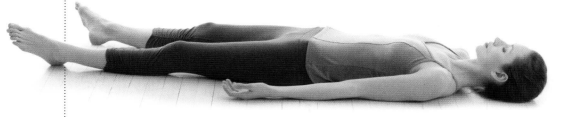

Bellows Breathing

Bellows breathing is a handy go-to practice that clears the nasal passages and also builds heat in the body, which releases stress, tension, and toxins from the system.

the ROUTINE

You can practice deep breathing anytime, including while you are practicing yoga.

Sit in a chair or on the floor, palms on your thighs. Close your eyes and take 3 deep inhales and exhales through your nose, keeping your mouth closed. /// Gradually increase the speed of your inhales and exhales until your breaths become short and fast. You will feel your stomach pressing in toward your spine on each exhale. Focus on sharp, full exhales. Your inhales will happen automatically between exhales, as you release your stomach. /// Once you are breathing at a very rapid rate try to sustain it for about 1 minute. Then, slowly lengthen your inhales and exhales until they return to long, deep breaths. Continue for another minute.

Alternate Nostril Breathing

Alternate nostril breathing is a meditative practice that switches breath between the two nostrils. We naturally alternate breath between each nostril every 2 to 3 hours. Alternate nostril breathing also increases digestive power, soothes and invigorates the nerves, clears the sinuses, alleviates headaches, promotes deep relaxation, and balances wake and sleep cycles.

the ROUTINE

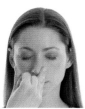

This practice produces optimal function of both sides of the brain and calms the mind and nervous system.

Sit in a comfortable position. Curl the forefinger and middle finger of your right hand into your palm. Place your right hand around your nose so your ring and pinkie fingers are alongside your left nostril. //// Close your left nostril with your ring finger and inhale slowly through your right nostril for 4 counts. Close the right nostril with your right thumb so both nostrils are closed and hold your breath for 4 counts. /// Release your ring finger and slowly exhale through your left nostril for 4 counts. /// Rest with all the air out of your lungs for 4 counts. /// With your thumb in the same position, inhale through your left nostril for 4 counts. Then close it and hold for 4 counts. /// Release your thumb and exhale through your right nostril for 4 counts. Then inhale through it for 4 counts. /// Hold and repeat the exhale/inhale on the left side. Continue for 5 minutes. If holding your breath for 4 counts is tough, start with 2 and build from there.

Breath of Fire

Breath of fire is a technique used in kundalini yoga practices to cleanse and energize the body. Breath of fire is great to build heat and is often used in nonkundalini yoga classes to warm up the body quickly.

the ROUTINE

You can do this on its own to begin or end your meditation, or add it to your physical yoga practice to build heat.

Sit in a comfortable position. /// Close your eyes, rest your attention on your breath, and begin to take long, deep inhales and exhales. At the end of each exhale, squeeze all the air out. /// Slowly start to increase the rate of your inhales and exhales. You might sound like a steam engine, and you will notice your abdomen contracting each time you exhale. /// Keep increasing the speed until you are comfortable with maintaining a steady fast pace for a minute. Focus on even and sharp inhales and exhales. /// To come out of the breath of fire, gradually slow down your breathing until you're back to your long, deep breathing.

clear your mind *with* **meditation**

To practice yoga effectively—and to achieve any of its benefits—you need to clear your mind of clutter. As the Indian mystic Osho once said, "Silence is the space in which one awakens, and the noisy mind is the space in which one remains asleep. If your mind continues chattering, you are asleep."

In yoga, meditation is the practice of resting your attention on your breath instead of getting wrapped up in the ongoing drama of your thoughts. Once your thoughts settle, your mind is free from all the clutter that keeps you busy and restless and unable to make good decisions. This isn't just one of those intuitive things. There's hard physical evidence that meditation can reprogram your brain to work more effectively.

In his research on people who meditate regularly, Richard Davidson, PhD, a neurologist at the University of Wisconsin, found that experienced meditators produce more gamma brain waves, the kind that are associated with intense, clear thinking. And the more you meditate, the more benefit you enjoy.

There's also reason to believe that meditation slows brain aging. Researchers at Massachusetts General Hospital did MRI scans on the brains of people who meditated regularly and found that their prefrontal cortices (responsible for attention and sensory perception) didn't show typical age-related thinning.

As for shorter-term effects, wouldn't you like to simply feel more refreshed during the day? You could nap, I suppose, but midday snoozes have nothing on meditation when it comes to keeping you alert. Researchers at the University of Kentucky tested people's reaction times before and after 40 minutes of sleeping, reading, talking, or meditating. Turns out, meditation was the only activity that led to an immediate improvement in performance.

You won't need to om like a Tibetan monk to enjoy the benefits of meditation. You can start slowly, fitting 5 minutes into your day here and there, and eventually work up to longer practices when you have the time.

You can meditate sitting or lying down, during physical yoga practice or not. You can even practice meditation while you're waiting in line at the grocery store or making dinner. Just a few minutes of shifting your attention away from your thoughts and to your breath helps calm your mind, refocus your energy, and revitalize your entire system. It doesn't take much to put you back in touch with you. Some quick practice can make all the difference.

On the following page is a meditation technique borrowed from kundalini yoga to help you explore the connection between your mind and your body. (You'll also find additional meditations built into the yoga sequences throughout the book.)

You'll be sitting in a comfortable position, holding your arms up in a V shape. Before you start to think this is easy and wonder what the point of holding up your arms is, rest assured that this exercise will prove how much power your mind has. You are strong enough physically to hold your arms up for several minutes. Your mind might try to tell you otherwise, especially as the seconds tick by. This meditation teaches you that you can either pay attention to your breathing, relax, and use the least amount of effort to stay in the pose, or you can allow your thoughts to distract you, hold on to tension, and fight to stay in the pose.

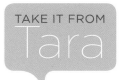

WHAT IS A MANTRA?

A mantra is a word or phrase, repeated silently in the mind or spoken, that helps set an intention with the purpose of transformation. Mantras originated in India's Vedic tradition, an ancient spiritual and mystical tradition that teaches how to live a virtuous life. They're also a part of Hindu and Buddhist traditions. A mantra can vary from a passage of classical scripture to a personalized hope or desire. You can choose your own mantra to help solidify and maintain focus on your intention. Mantras are often aligned with the breath: Inhale worthiness; exhale obstacles. Shanti is the most common mantra you may hear. It means "peace" in our thoughts and actions toward ourselves and others.

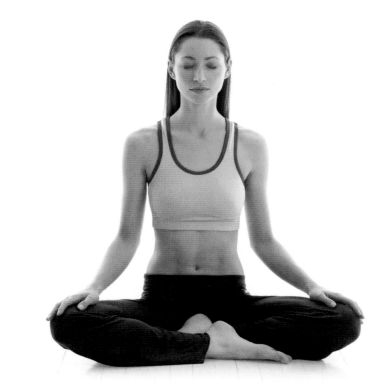

◾ *Seated Meditation*

Sit up tall on the floor in a comfortable position. If you like, you can try sitting on a block or a rolled-up towel and folding your legs in so your knees relax out to the sides. (The block gives your hips and spine a chance to sit up straight without stress on your lower back.) Relax your shoulders and rest your palms on your thighs. Close your eyes and rest your attention on your breath. Inhale deeply for 4 counts then exhale for 4 counts. Repeat 10 times, then return to normal breathing.

◾ *Seated Meditation, Arms in V*

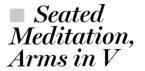

Reach your arms up so they form a V, keeping your shoulders relaxed. Close your eyes and stay here for 5 minutes.

If 5 minutes seems like an eternity, start by holding your arms up for just 1 minute. Do that three times a week for 1 week, then try for 2 minutes in each attempt the following week. Add a minute each day from there, and see if you can build up to 10 minutes.

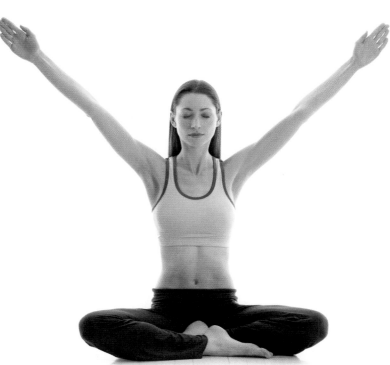

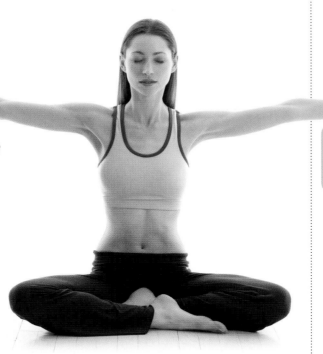

Seated Meditation, Arms Out to Sides

After you've held your arms up in a V, lower them until they're parallel to the floor, and press your palms straight out to the sides. Hold for 10 inhales and exhales. Then close your fingers into fists and flick your fingers outward. Repeat 10 times, then slowly lower your arms to your lap. Stay here for 10 deep breaths.

Sage Secrets | QUIET YOUR THOUGHTS

THE BUDDHA SAID that we suffer in life because we are trapped in our minds. When you can free your mind by first gaining control over your thoughts and then by emptying your mind of all the constant thinking, then you are free from suffering.

Many problems we face in our lives are products of our thinking. While our lives are always taking place right here in this current moment, our thinking is always drawn to rethinking what has already happened and looking ahead to what might happen. This worry creates fears and insecurities, and keeps us from being fully right where we are.

If you can quiet some of this constant reflection and projection, you can gain an incredible amount of freedom to experience what is actually happening right in front of you. Meditating helps you get there by teaching you to take a step back from your thoughts and make choices that are healthy, without the limitations of what was or might someday be.

align your body

Alignment is key to an efficient yoga practice. Proper body alignment is all about stacking your bones so your muscles and circulation can work effectively. When your body is in the correct position, you get the most benefit out of each pose.

The more you practice yoga, the better you'll be able to sense your alignment and make automatic fixes. You'll start to notice how you feel in the poses and find subtle ways to adjust. But don't overthink it! Yoga is designed to put you in tune with your physical, mental, and spiritual states of being. It's easy to get so consumed with alignment that you lose touch with those senses and don't derive as much benefit from your practice.

Here's how to line up your body—and mind—to get the most from each pose.

■ **TAKE A DEEP BREATH.** You'll need to slow down and deepen your breathing to get the most benefit from the poses. Whenever you notice yourself breathing short and fast, guide your breath back to long and deep.
Try it: Start by practicing a 4-count long, deep breath. Wherever you are right now, take a deep breath through your nose. Exhale all the air out. Then inhale starting from your belly and count 1, move up through your ribs and count 2, 3, and finally through your upper chest and count 4. Hold for 2 counts and slowly exhale. Nice, right?

■ **FOCUS YOUR MIND.** Alignment doesn't stop with the body. When your mind is in the right place, everything else falls into position. Keeping your mental focus sharp and reining in wandering thoughts is essential.
Try it: Try setting an intention—or focus—for yourself each time you practice. An example of an intention is "I will try to focus on my breath instead of my thoughts during the whole class. This will help me focus in my life and control impulses so I can reach my weight-loss goal." It sets a mood for your practice that keeps you on target.

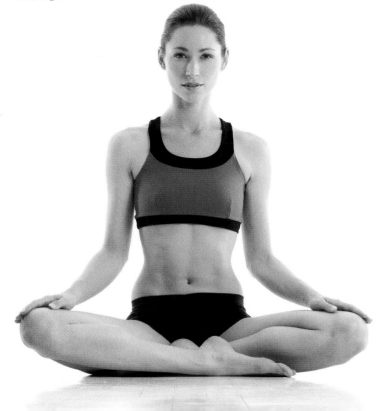

■**KEEP YOUR ELBOWS SLIGHTLY BENT.** Locking your elbows during weight-bearing poses such as plank and down dog is another recipe for wrist and shoulder injury. This is especially the case if your elbows tend to hyperextend. Aim to keep your arms slightly bent (they'll be closer to straight than you think) and you'll get strong and toned even faster.

Try it: Come to all fours. Spread your fingers and bend your elbows out to the sides. Slowly start to straighten your arms, and stop when your upper arms and forearms are in a straight line. If you hyperextend naturally, they'll feel bent but will actually be straight.

■**SPREAD YOUR FINGERS.** Many poses—plank, down dog, handstand—place your weight on your arms, so it's important to have a solid base. Spreading your fingers helps build strength by engaging your arms and shoulders; weak, passive fingers can overstress your wrists and shoulders, leading to injury.

Try it: Practice spreading your fingers while doing a common pose like down dog: Come to all fours with your knees under your hips and hands under your shoulders. Bend your elbows slightly and spread your fingers as if you were digging into wet sand. Straighten your arms, keeping your fingers spread wide. Tuck your toes under, lift your hips, and extend your legs. Press your shoulders toward the floor and relax your neck. Press your palms against the floor a few inches in front of your feet. Walk your feet back, lift your hips, and press your heels toward the floor. Relax your shoulders and head.

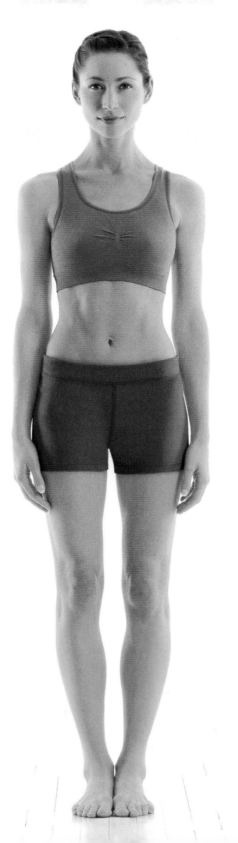

■ **KEEP YOUR FEET UNDER YOUR HIPS.** Take notice of your foot placement habits in standing poses. You are the most efficient when your feet are directly under your hip bones and your heels are aligned behind your toes.

Try it: Stand naturally at the front of your mat. Now take a look at your feet. See if they are set wider or narrower than your hip bones. Are your toes pointing out or in, or straight forward? Make sure your feet are parallel to each other. They can be together or slightly apart.

essential
poses

Master these moves for a
sound body and mind

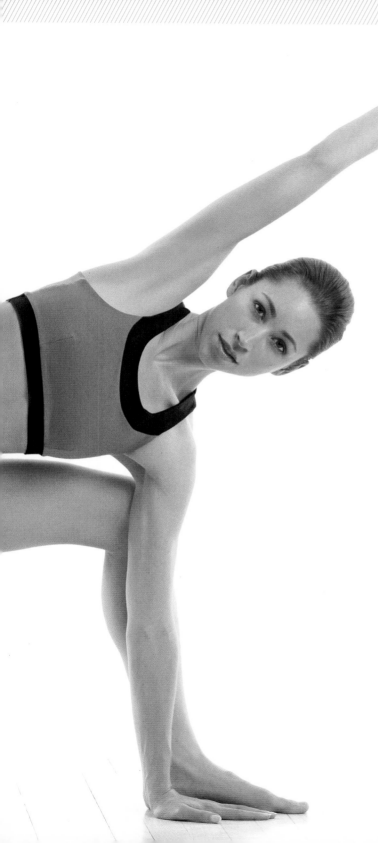

In this chapter,

you'll find a how-to primer on every single pose that makes up the 15-minute routines throughout the rest of the book. To keep things simple, they are divided into categories as follows: Standing Poses; Seated Poses; Arm Balances and Inversions; and Other Poses (Lying-Down Poses, Back Bends, and Partner-Supported Poses).

Within each category, specific moves are designated as Main Poses. Master these basic versions and you'll be able to do all their variations with superior form—and get the most benefits. In some cases, there is no Main Pose; instead, I'll give you a sequence for achieving a pose that may take you some time to get good at, such as a headstand or handstand. Pay close attention to the alignment tips on every page—the better your form, the better your yoga.

The pictures here are for basic reference. Even when a pose is shown from just one side (with the right leg forward, for example), you'll need to practice it on both sides to work your body evenly. But later in the book, when you start practicing the 15-minute routines, I'll give you specific directions for when to switch sides and how long to hold each pose. So roll out your mats. It's time to make the yoga!

standing poses

Standing poses build strength, confidence, and total-body awareness. They sculpt and tone your entire body, leaving you with a strong, sexy shape and full of energy. When you perform the poses in correct alignment, your body develops strength and flexibility evenly. When you breathe deeply in the poses, you get the most benefits physically and mentally. You have your whole life to practice, so start where you are and build from there.

Main POSE

Standing

Stand with your feet together and your heels directly behind your toes. Engage your quads, spread your toes, and relax your arms down by your sides.

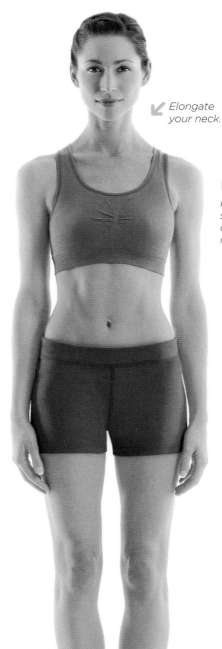

Elongate your neck.

Keep your shoulders down and relaxed.

Sometimes the simple act of standing can reveal so much about you. Take the time to stand up straight, head high, projecting confidence for 20 long, deep breaths.

Keep your feet parallel.

■ *Standing Arm Reach*

Inhale and extend your arms overhead. Lengthen through your sides and relax your shoulders. Look up toward your hands.

■ *Standing Side Opener*

Raise your arms over your head and grab your right wrist with your left hand. Bend sideways from your waist to the left side.

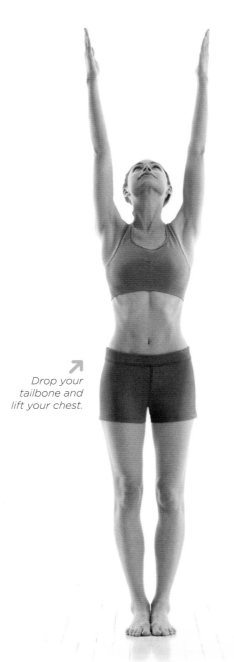

Drop your tailbone and lift your chest.

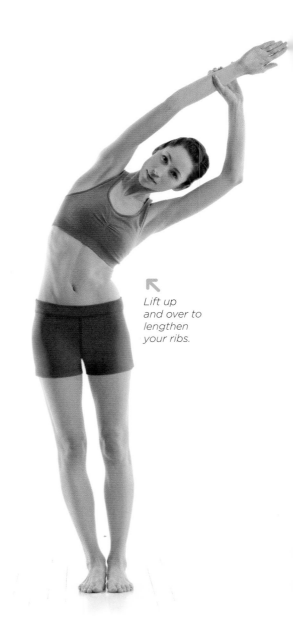

Lift up and over to lengthen your ribs.

Standing Palm Press

Lace your fingers together and press your palms up toward the ceiling, lengthening your arms.

Standing Arch

Press your thumbs to your lower back. Bring your shoulder blades together, arch your back, and press your chest straight up.

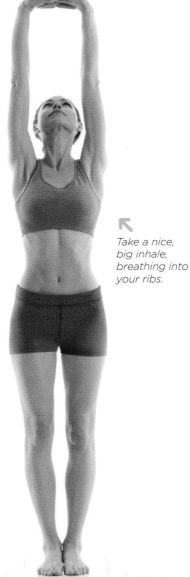

Look up at your fingers and relax your shoulders.

Take a nice, big inhale, breathing into your ribs.

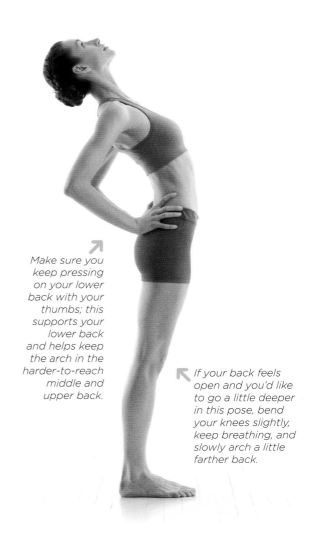

Make sure you keep pressing on your lower back with your thumbs; this supports your lower back and helps keep the arch in the harder-to-reach middle and upper back.

If your back feels open and you'd like to go a little deeper in this pose, bend your knees slightly, keep breathing, and slowly arch a little farther back.

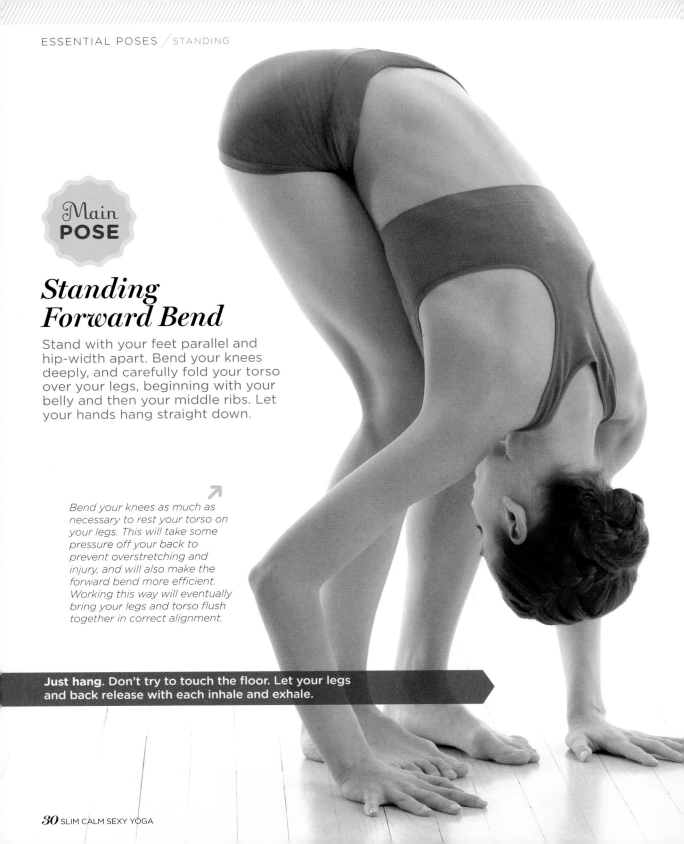

Main
POSE

Standing Forward Bend

Stand with your feet parallel and hip-width apart. Bend your knees deeply, and carefully fold your torso over your legs, beginning with your belly and then your middle ribs. Let your hands hang straight down.

Bend your knees as much as necessary to rest your torso on your legs. This will take some pressure off your back to prevent overstretching and injury, and will also make the forward bend more efficient. Working this way will eventually bring your legs and torso flush together in correct alignment.

Just hang. Don't try to touch the floor. Let your legs and back release with each inhale and exhale.

◼ *Standing Forward Bend, Elbow Hold*

Grab your elbows and let your head hang heavy.

Make sure your weight is evenly distributed on your feet. Doing so helps to strengthen and release your muscles correctly. When standing, we often favor one leg, or rock to our heels or toes instead of standing equally centered on both feet. You can check this in your forward bend. If your hips are behind you and you feel as if you are locking your knees, you probably have too much weight on your heels. Bring your hips forward over your feet and your weight will be evenly distributed.

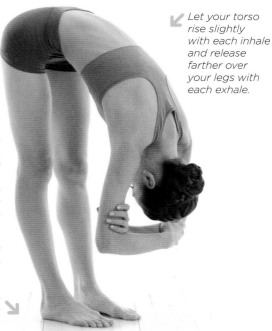

Let your torso rise slightly with each inhale and release farther over your legs with each exhale.

◼ *Standing Forward Bend, Neck Release*

Lace your fingers together at the base of your neck and gently guide the top of your head toward the floor.

Placing your feet hip-width apart usually leaves about the width of two fists between them. You can check this by making fists and placing them side by side between your feet. When your feet are under your hip bones, you are balanced and able to build strength, release tension, and move efficiently.

Exhale and release your torso closer to your legs.

Bend your knees slightly if it's more comfortable for you.

Inhale and expand your sides.

Standing Forward Bend, Calf Hold

Release your hands and grab your calves, bending your elbows slightly out to the sides.

Back Lengthener with Easy Twist

Plant the fingers of your left hand on the floor a few inches in front of your feet. Bend your left knee slightly, open your chest to the right, and extend your right arm upward. Look up at your right hand.

Release your torso toward your legs on each exhale. ↘

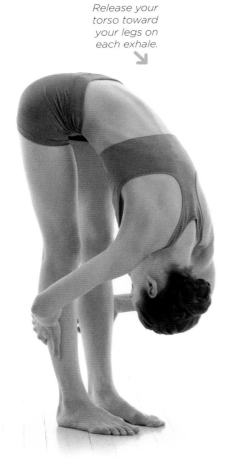

Lengthen your spine from your lower back out through the top of your head. ↘

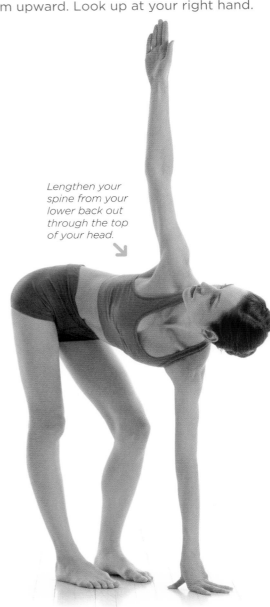

Standing Hand Step

Bend your knees, then gently step on both of your hands so that the tops of your hands are on the floor, fingers pointing behind you, and your toes are resting on the insides of your wrists. Keep your knees bent and breathe here for a few breaths. Let your head hang down.

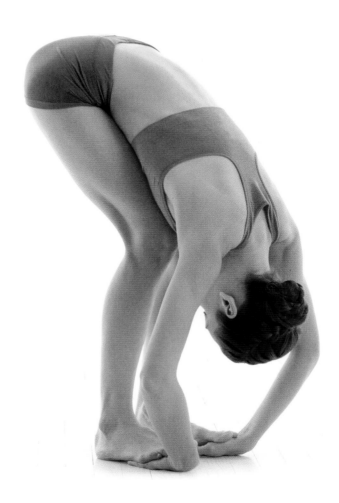

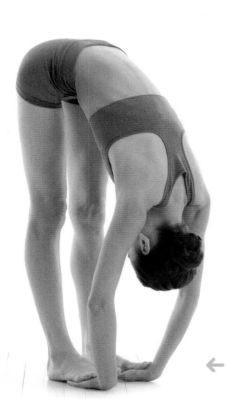

If your wrists feel good and the muscles in the backs of your thighs don't feel tight, try straightening your legs.

Main
POSE

Squat

Lower your body as far as you can by bending your knees and pushing your hips back. Point your toes out slightly and separate your feet as much as you need to in order to keep your heels on the floor. Lace your fingers together behind your head and let your head hang and your torso sink down between your legs.

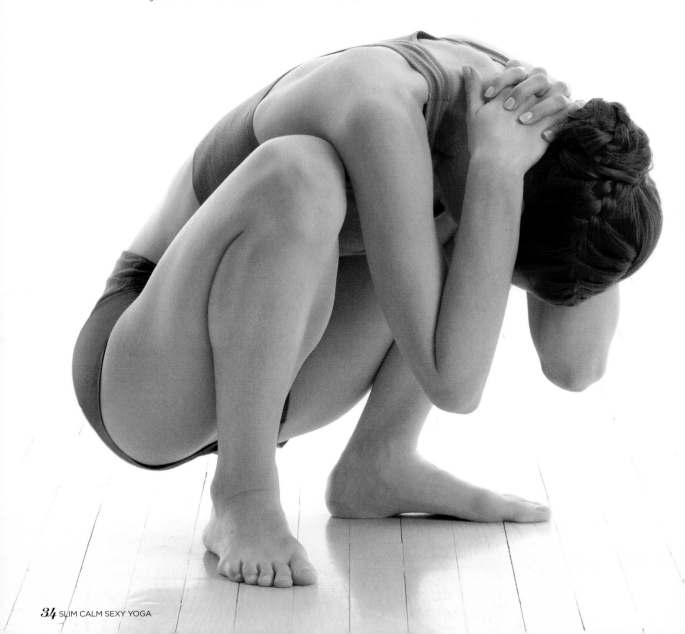

Squat Hang

Release your hands and place them on the floor in front of you, continuing to let your head and torso hang.

Squat Twist

Bring your left shoulder inside your left knee and rest your left hand on the floor. Press your right hand on your right thigh, just above your knee. Don't round your shoulders. Open your chest. Look up over your right shoulder.

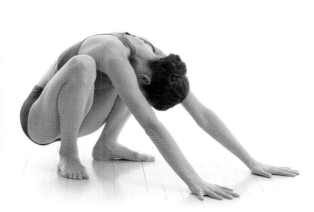

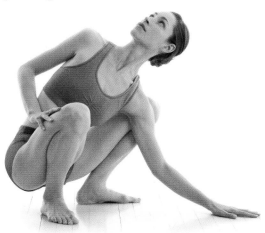

Squat Twist Bind

Wrap your right arm around and behind your back. Bring your left arm behind your left shin, and grab your right wrist with your left hand.

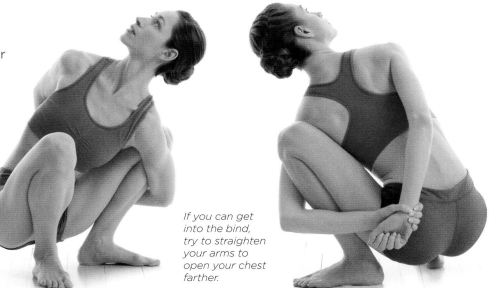

If you can get into the bind, try to straighten your arms to open your chest farther.

Down Dog

From standing, come down to all fours. Spread your fingers wide on your mat. Make sure your wrists are under your shoulders and your knees are under your hips. Tuck your toes, lift your hips up and back, and extend your legs. Press your shoulders toward the floor and relax your neck. Press your palms against the floor a few inches in front of your feet. Walk your feet back, lift your hips, and press your heels toward the floor. Relax your shoulders and head.

Spreading your fingers ensures a stable founda-tion that builds strength effectively and prevents injury. Whether you are on all fours or in plank, down dog, or handstand, spread your fingers wide, as if you were squishing them into wet sand.

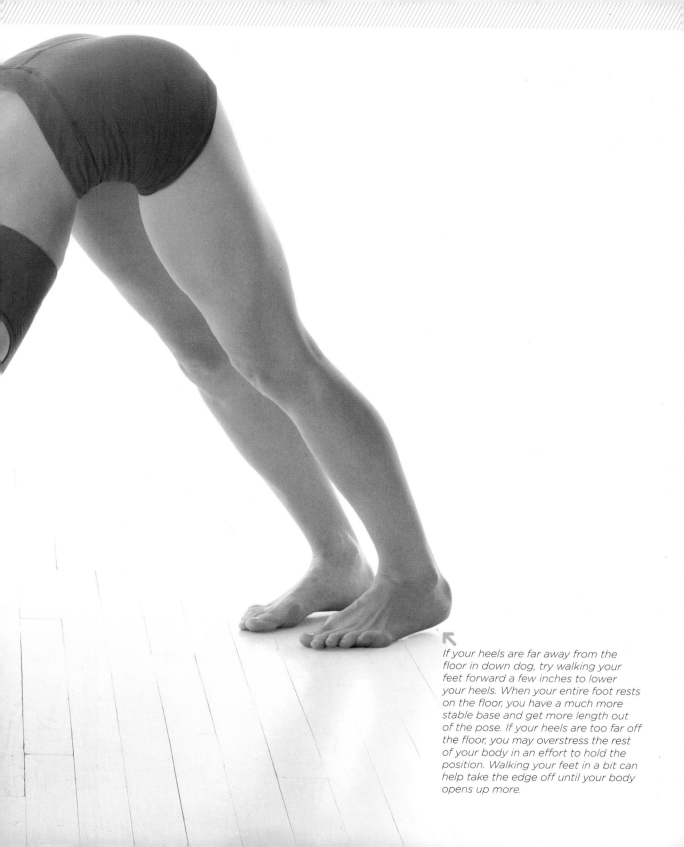

If your heels are far away from the floor in down dog, try walking your feet forward a few inches to lower your heels. When your entire foot rests on the floor, you have a much more stable base and get more length out of the pose. If your heels are too far off the floor, you may overstress the rest of your body in an effort to hold the position. Walking your feet in a bit can help take the edge off until your body opens up more.

Down Dog Split

Bring your right leg straight up behind you, foot flexed. Keep your hips square to the floor.

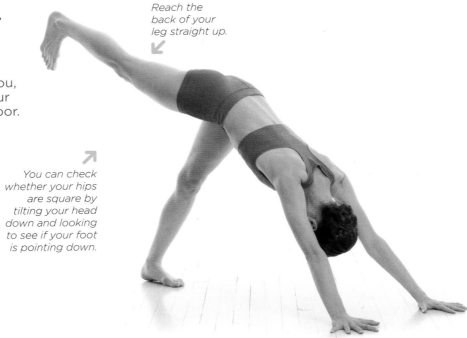

Reach the back of your leg straight up.

You can check whether your hips are square by tilting your head down and looking to see if your foot is pointing down.

Down Dog Split, Side Lift

Arc your right leg from behind you out to your right side so your toes point forward. Keep your right leg even with your hips, and keep both arms straight and strong.

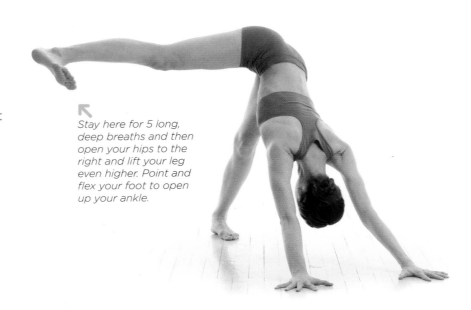

Stay here for 5 long, deep breaths and then open your hips to the right and lift your leg even higher. Point and flex your foot to open up your ankle.

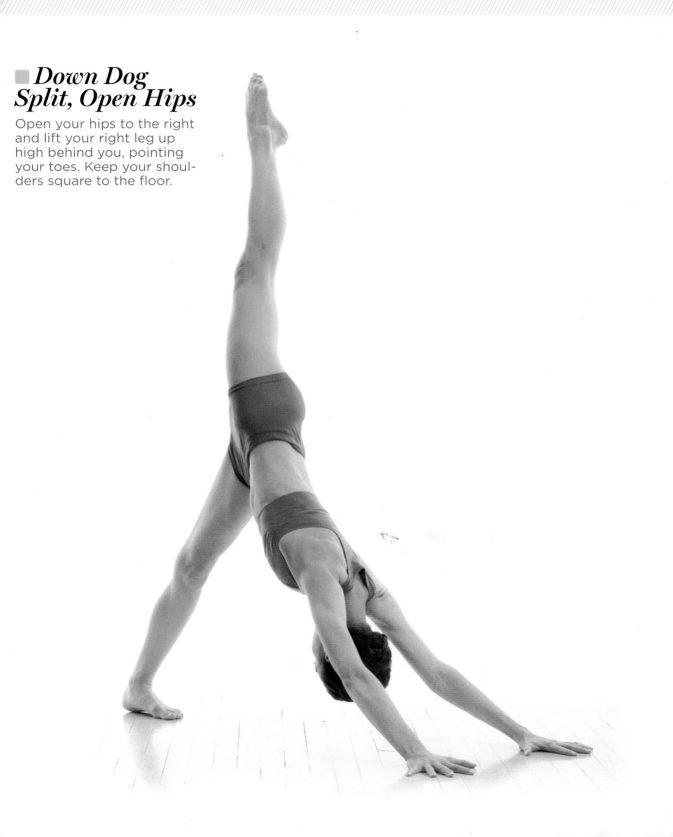

Down Dog Split, Open Hips

Open your hips to the right and lift your right leg up high behind you, pointing your toes. Keep your shoulders square to the floor.

■ *Down Dog Split, Open Hips and Shoulders*

Keeping your hips open to the right, open your shoulders to the right side.

■ *Down Dog Split, Forearm Lower*

Lower your left forearm to the floor.

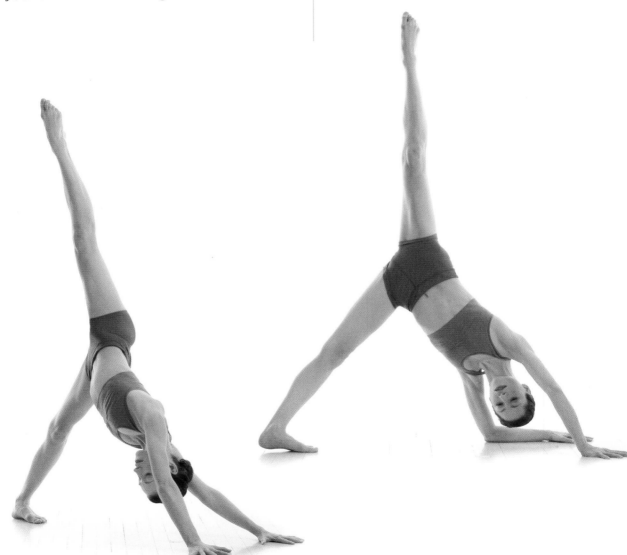

◼ *Down Dog, Hands on Chair*

Stand facing a chair. Make sure your heels are straight behind your toes and your feet are under your hips. Place your hands on the seat, and walk your feet back a few steps until your torso is nearly parallel to the floor and your arms are fully extended.

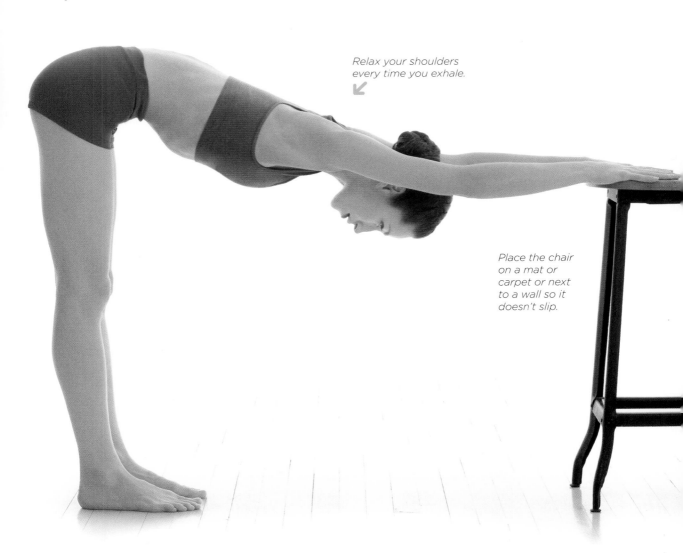

Relax your shoulders every time you exhale.

Place the chair on a mat or carpet or next to a wall so it doesn't slip.

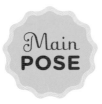

Main POSE

If this is difficult at first, try shifting your hips back toward your heels a little, bringing your shoulders from directly above to slightly behind your wrists. This will make it easier to maintain a slow, controlled motion.

↘

Palm Raise

Come to all fours. Make sure your hands are directly under your shoulders and your knees are under your hips. Spread your fingers wide and press your palms and fingers firmly against the floor. With a slow, continuous motion, raise and lower your palms 10 times.

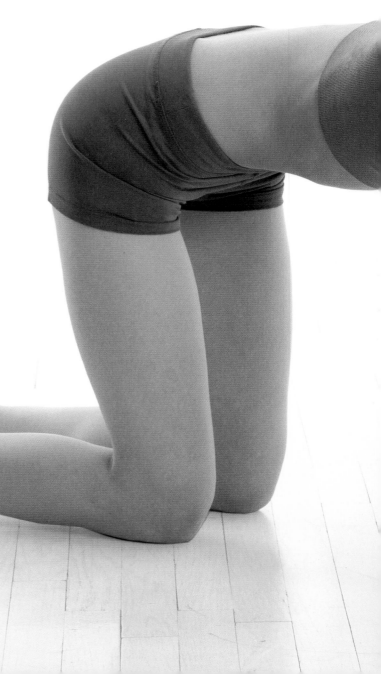

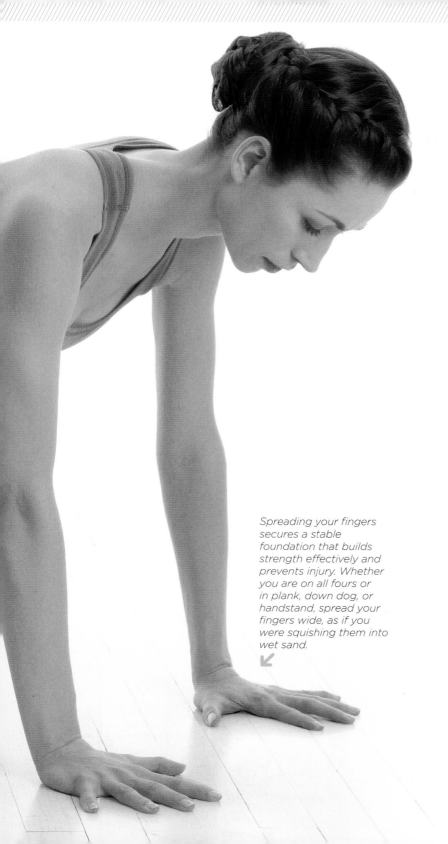

Spreading your fingers
secures a stable
foundation that builds
strength effectively and
prevents injury. Whether
you are on all fours or
in plank, down dog, or
handstand, spread your
fingers wide, as if you
were squishing them into
wet sand.
↙

VARIATION 1
Turn your fingers to
point slightly outward and
repeat the raises.

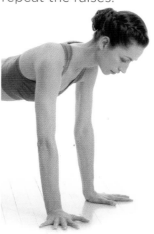

VARIATION 2
Now turn your fingers to
point slightly inward and
repeat the raises.

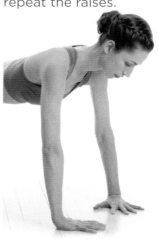

■ *Fists Facing*

Make fists with both hands. Bending your elbows out to the sides, place the tops of your hands on the floor so your fingers face each other. Start to straighten your arms, but only as much as you can while keeping your fists tight.

Hold the straightest wrist and forearm position you can while keeping your fists tight.

Wrist Release

Rest your palms on the floor so your fingers face forward and are spread evenly. Turn your right hand to the right until your fingers face your knees. Lower your palm to the floor. Gently lower your hips back toward your heels. Go only as far as you can without any pain; it might be enough just to keep your shoulders over your wrists.

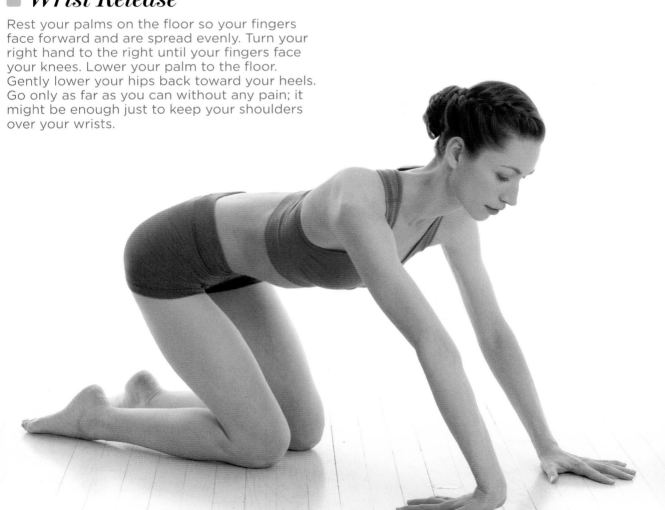

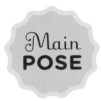

Main
POSE

Low Lunge

Step forward with your right foot. Press your fingertips on the floor, with one hand on each side of your right foot. Bend your knees slightly and step back with your left leg into a long, low lunge. Your right leg should be bent deeply and your left leg should be straight.

Reach out through your left heel and sink your hips low.

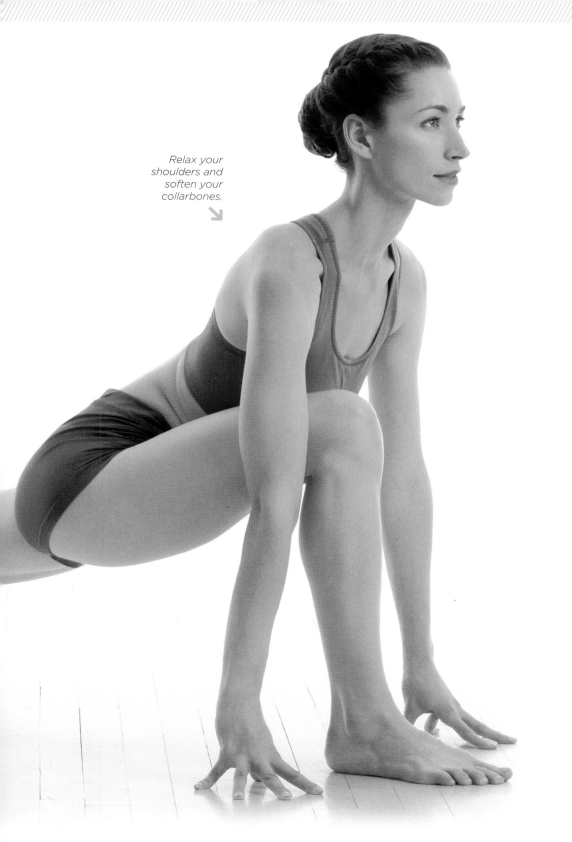

Relax your shoulders and soften your collarbones.

■ *Low Lunge, Back Knee Down, Hands on Front Knee*

Gently lower your left knee to the floor. Place your hands on top of your right knee and bring your shoulder blades together. Sink your hips forward.

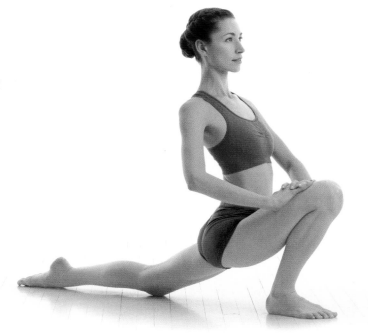

■ *Low Lunge, Back Knee Down, with Twist, Hip Hold*

Bring your left hand to your right knee and wrap your right arm around your back so you can hold your left hip with your hand. Pull your left hip up to square your hips and bring your right shin perpendicular to the floor. Twist your torso around to the right.

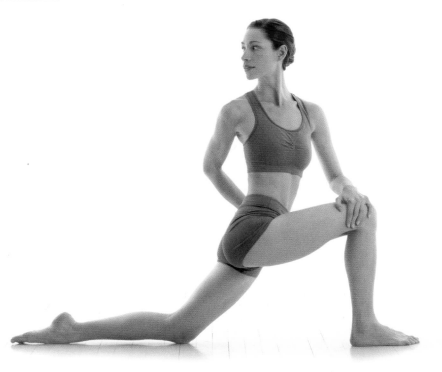

Low Lunge, Back Knee Down, Palm Press

Lace your fingers together, press your palms up, and lengthen your arms. Look up at your fingers and relax your shoulders down as you sink your hips forward.

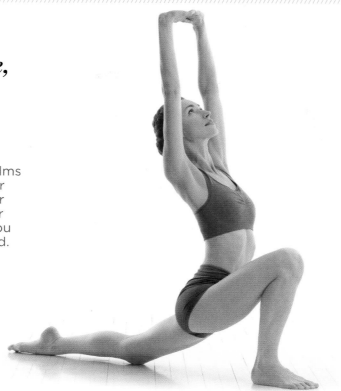

Low Lunge, Back Knee Down, Hip Release (Lizard)

Bring your hands down on each side of your right foot. Move your right foot toward your right hand or the right edge of your mat. Point your toes forward and make sure your heel is directly behind your toes. Bring your forearms to the floor inside your right foot. Lengthen your chest forward with each inhale, and sink your hips and chest closer to the floor with each exhale.

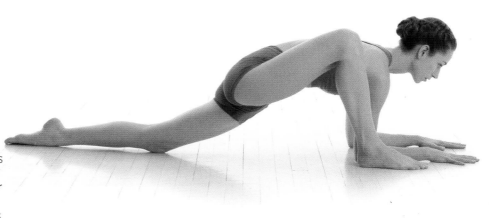

◼ *Low Lunge, Sit on Back Heel, Forward Bend*

Move your hips back and rest your weight on your left heel. Extend your right leg in front of you, resting your heel on the floor, foot flexed. Rest your fingertips on the floor on each side of your knees. Inhale, bend at the waist, and lengthen your back. Exhale and twist over your right leg.

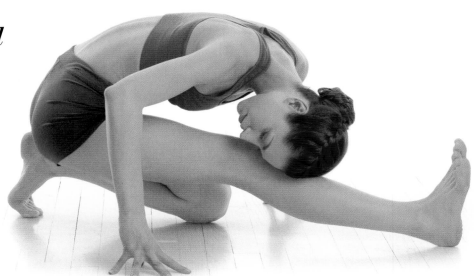

◼ *High Lunge*

Bend your right knee over your right foot so your thigh is parallel to the floor. Extend your arms straight up over your ears. Sink your hips and relax your shoulders. Put some weight onto your left foot, reaching your heel out behind you for stability.

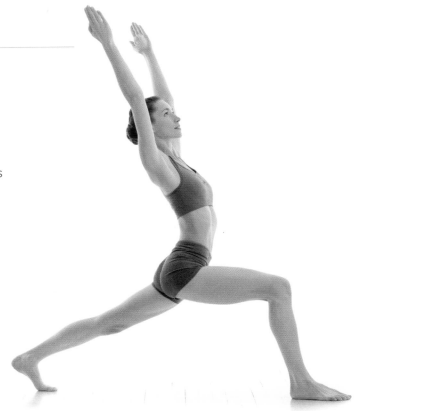

High Lunge with Twist

Reach your left arm forward and your right arm back and open your torso to your right side. Make sure your shoulders are over your hips. Relax your shoulders and look back over your right hand.

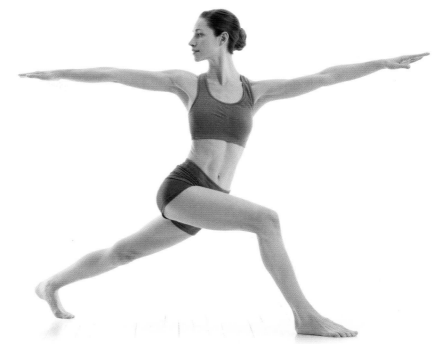

High Lunge with Twist, Fingertips Down

Lower your left arm along the outside of your right knee and touch your fingertips to the floor. Extend your right arm upward, relax your shoulders, and look up over your right hand.

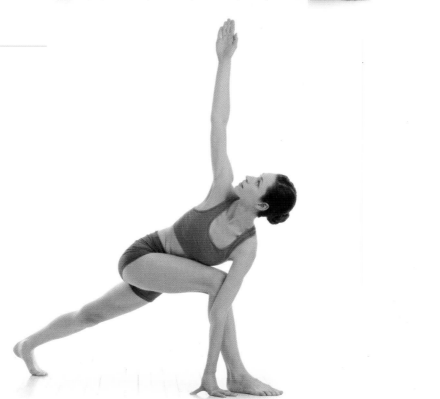

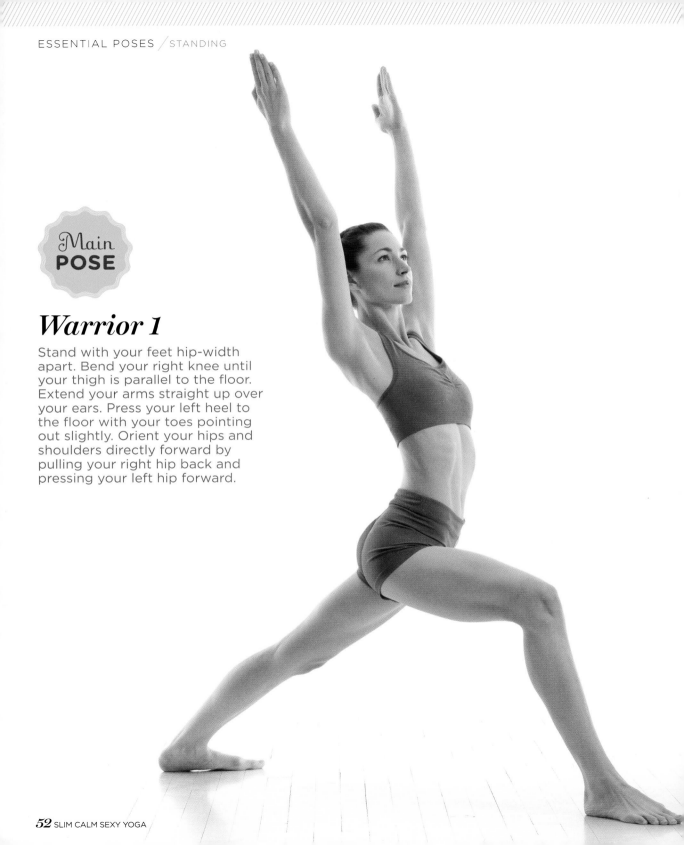

Main
POSE

Warrior 1

Stand with your feet hip-width apart. Bend your right knee until your thigh is parallel to the floor. Extend your arms straight up over your ears. Press your left heel to the floor with your toes pointing out slightly. Orient your hips and shoulders directly forward by pulling your right hip back and pressing your left hip forward.

Warrior 1, Interlaced Hands, Shoulder Release

Lower your arms down by your sides. Lace your fingers together behind your back and inhale to lift your chest up. Exhale and fold your torso inside your right leg, lowering the top of your head toward the floor. Relax your shoulders and reach your arms up behind you.

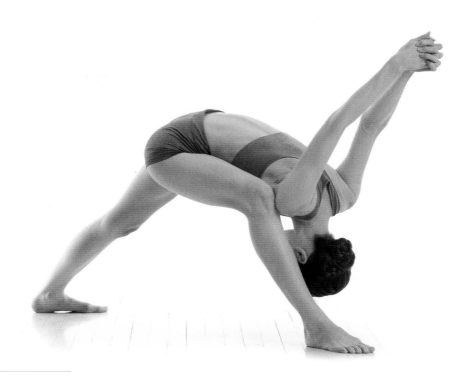

Warrior 2

Open your hips and shoulders to face your left side. Extend your right arm forward and your left arm back so they are parallel to the floor. Focus your gaze over your right hand.

Reach out evenly forward and back through your arms and fingertips.

Lengthen your spine as you sink your hips low.

Press through the outside edge of your left foot.

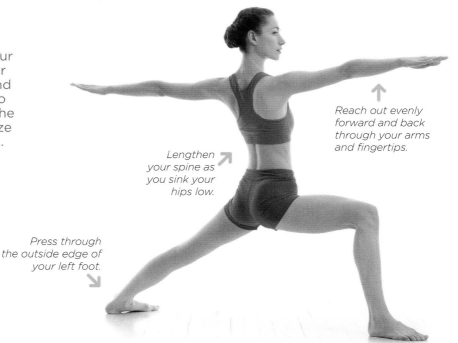

Warrior 3

Bend at the hips and lengthen your torso forward so it's parallel to the floor, reaching your arms straight forward past your ears. Shift your weight onto your right leg and lift your hips, raising your left leg until it's parallel to the floor. Flex your left foot.

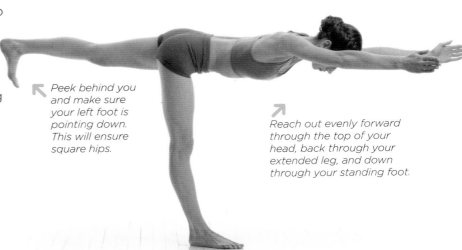

Peek behind you and make sure your left foot is pointing down. This will ensure square hips.

Reach out evenly forward through the top of your head, back through your extended leg, and down through your standing foot.

Warrior 3, Fingertips on Floor

Lower your arms and press your fingertips against the floor a few inches in front of your right foot.

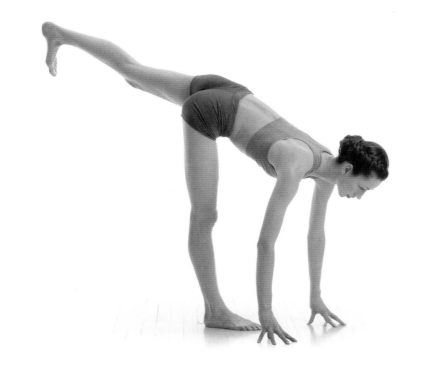

Warrior 3, Hands on Shin

Lift your fingertips off the floor and bring your hands up to the front of your right shin.

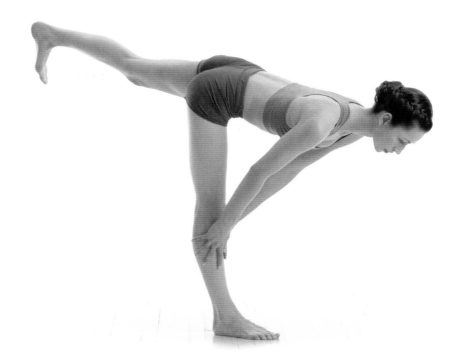

Peaceful Warrior

Lower your left leg to the floor. Keeping your hips low, bring your left arm down to the outside of your left calf and extend your right arm straight up. Look up toward your right hand.

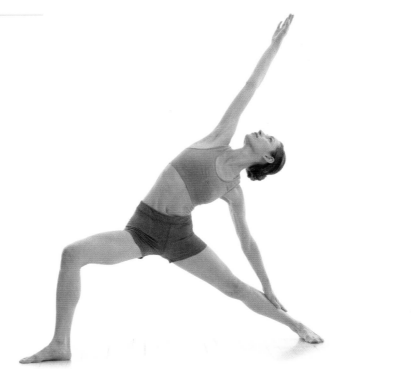

Main
POSE

Triangle

Come into a low lunge, pointing your left foot forward and your right foot out to the side. Open your hips and shoulders to face your right side, and straighten your left leg. Extend your left arm forward and your right arm back. Leading with the left side of your ribs, bring your shoulders out over your left leg and either place your left hand on your left shin or press your fingertips to the mat outside of your left foot. Extend your right arm straight up. Open your torso to the right and look up toward your right hand.

Triangle with Block

Grab a block and place it on the floor close to your left foot. Press firmly into the block with your left hand. Extend your right arm straight up above your shoulders and look toward your right hand.

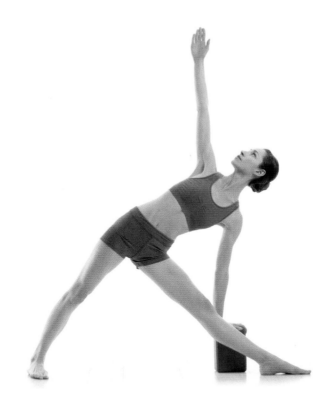

Rotated Triangle

Bring the fingertips of your right hand to the floor outside your left foot. Open your shoulders to the left and extend your left arm straight up. Bring your right foot forward about a foot and press your heel down so your toes point a little out to your right side. Square your hips by pulling your left hip back and your right hip forward.

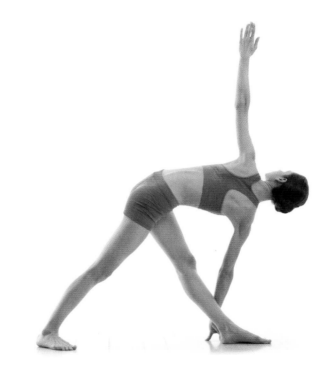

▪ *Extended Side Angle*

Gently bring the finger-tips of your left hand to the floor inside your left foot. Turn your torso toward the right and reach your right arm forward past your ear. Push down on your left hand and continue to rotate your shoulders and torso to the right. Look toward your right palm.

Lengthen and breathe into both sides. ↘

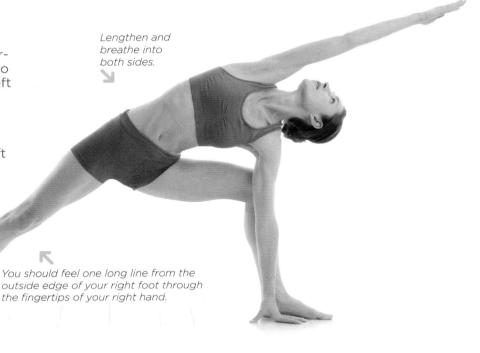

You should feel one long line from the outside edge of your right foot through the fingertips of your right hand. ↖

▪ *Extended Side Angle with Block*

Place a block on the floor inside your left foot and rest your left hand on it. Reach your right arm forward past your ear and open your torso from your belly up through your shoulders. Look toward your right palm.

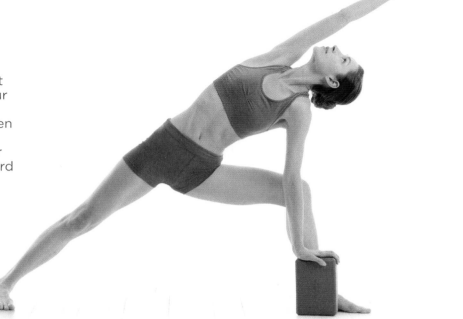

Bound Extended Side Angle

Wrap your right arm around your back and bring your left arm under your left thigh. Join hands and open your torso to the right. Turn your head to the right and reach the top of your head forward. Lift your torso away from your thigh.

Single-Leg Forward Bend with Blocks

Stand with your right foot about 2 feet in front of your left foot. Place a block on each side of your right foot. Carefully place each hand on a block. Pull your right hip back so both hips are square to the front. With both legs straight, bend at the waist.

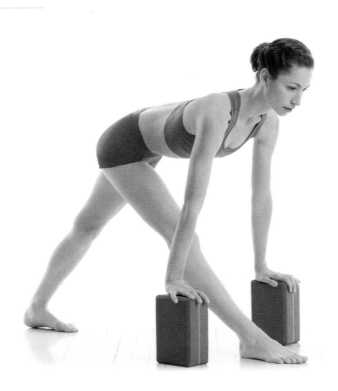

Single-Leg Forward Bend

Move the blocks aside and place your fingertips on the floor on each side of your right foot, elbows slightly bent. Hang your torso over your right leg.

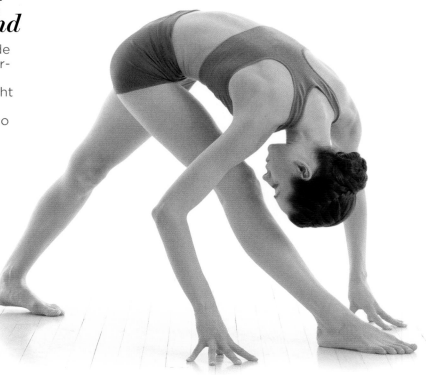

GET MORE STRETCH

Guide your right hip back to square your hips in single-leg forward bend. Working with square hips in this pose allows your body to effectively release tension and create flexibility in the hamstring.

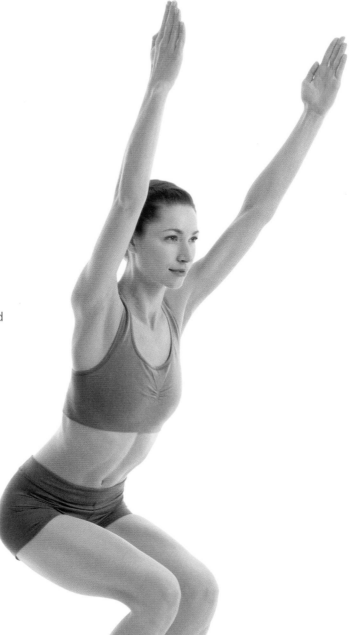

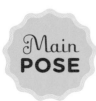

Chair

Stand with your feet under your
hips. Bend your knees deeply and
extend your arms overhead.

Try to keep a straight back. It's easy to arch your lower back as you reach higher with your arms and chest. To take the arch out of your lower back, pull your lower belly in and tuck your tailbone.

▪ *Tree*

Straighten your legs and grab your right ankle with your right hand. Press the sole of your right foot into your left upper thigh. When you feel steady, extend your arms overhead.

▪ *Standing Split*

Bring your fingertips to the floor, with one hand on either side of each foot. Lift your left leg back as high as you can, pointing your toes. Release your head toward your shin.

Reaching out evenly in all directions helps with balance. Imagine a string is pulling your left foot up while a magnet is pulling your right foot down. →

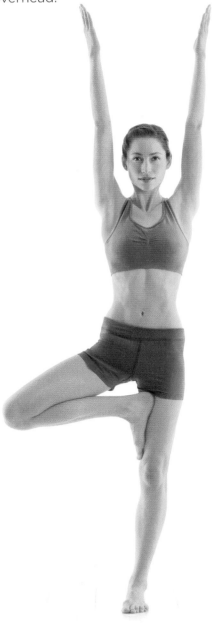

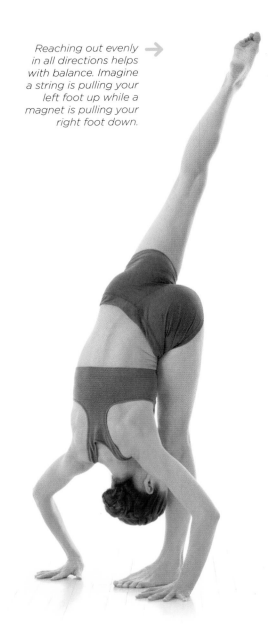

Standing Split Squat

Inhale as you bend both knees, lower your hips toward the floor, and bring your left knee outside your right ankle. Hover a few inches above the ground with your left shin parallel to the floor, toes pointed.

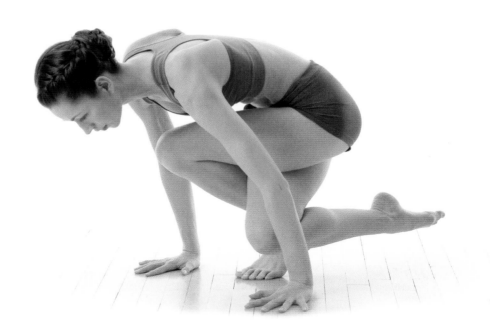

Standing Twisted Leg Extension

Return to standing. Bend your right knee to your chest and grab the outside of your right foot with your left hand. Lengthen out of your lower back and extend your right leg forward. Open your torso toward the right and extend your right arm behind you, parallel to the floor. Look toward your right hand.

Press firmly down through your standing leg by spreading your toes, engaging all the muscles in your leg, and pushing your foot into the floor. You may hear in yoga class to "push the floor away." That's what the teacher is talking about. ↘

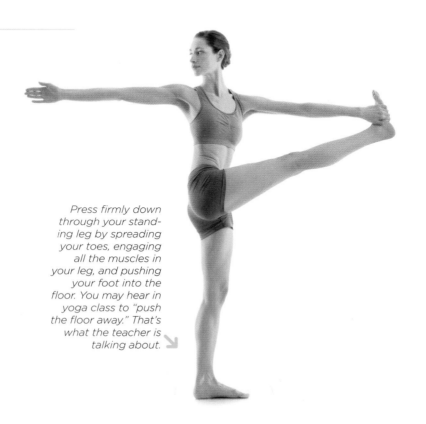

Standing Shin Hug

Lift your right leg and bend your knee in to your chest; you can bend your left leg slightly for balance. Wrap your hands around your right shin and hug your knee to your chest.

Big-Toe Hold, Front

Bring the forefinger and middle finger of your right hand around your right big toe. Rest your left hand on your left hip for balance. Lengthen your back and straighten your left leg. If your back is straight and your left leg is also straight, try extending your right leg forward.

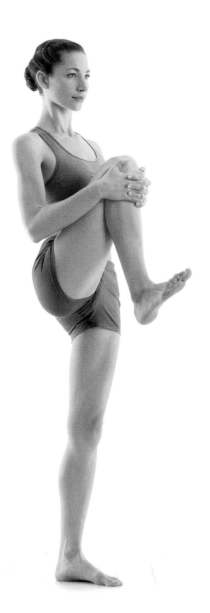

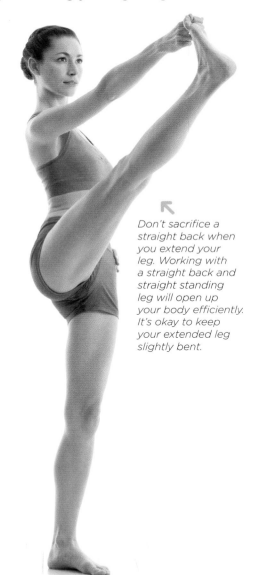

Don't sacrifice a straight back when you extend your leg. Working with a straight back and straight standing leg will open up your body efficiently. It's okay to keep your extended leg slightly bent.

Big-Toe Hold, Side

Keeping the big-toe hold, extend your right leg out to your right side.

Dancer

Come back to your shin hug and grab the inside of your right shin (or ankle) with your right hand. Raise your right leg as high as you can behind you while continuing to hold your shin with your right hand. Reach your left arm up to counterbalance.

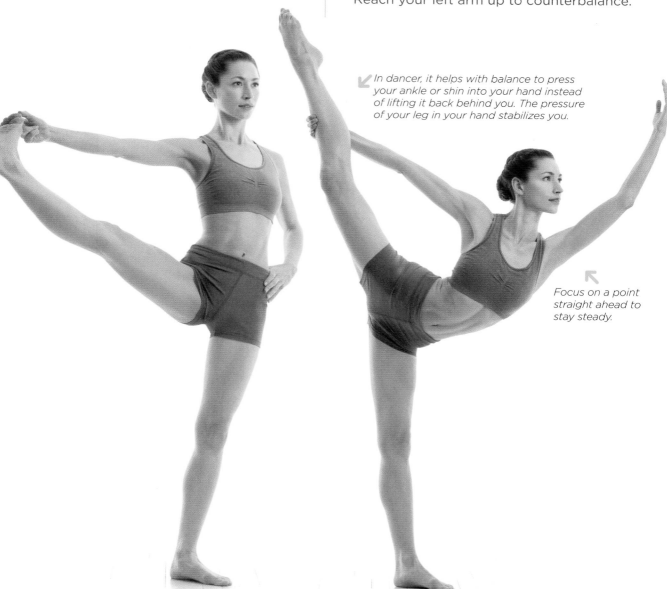

In dancer, it helps with balance to press your ankle or shin into your hand instead of lifting it back behind you. The pressure of your leg in your hand stabilizes you.

Focus on a point straight ahead to stay steady.

Half Moon

Bend at the waist and place the fingertips of your right hand on the floor a few inches in front of your right foot. Straighten your legs and lift your left leg straight behind you, flexing your foot. Open your hips, torso, and shoulders to the left and bring your left arm straight up. Look toward your left hand.

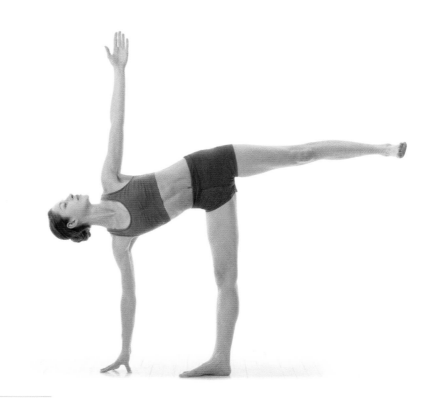

Twisted Half Moon

Stay on your right foot and bring the finger-tips of your left hand to the floor under your left shoulder. Square off your hips, then open your torso and shoulder to the right and lift your right arm straight up.

You can check to see if your hips are square by dropping your head and making sure your left foot is pointing down.

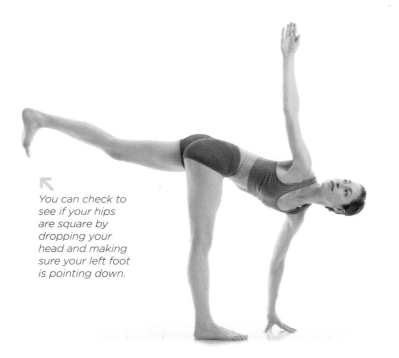

Half Moon, Bent Knee, Arch

Twist your torso to the left, rest the fingertips of your right hand on the floor, and raise your left hand off the floor. Bend your left knee and grab the top of your left foot with your left hand. Gently pull your left foot back behind your hips so your bent knee points to the right, open your chest, and look up.

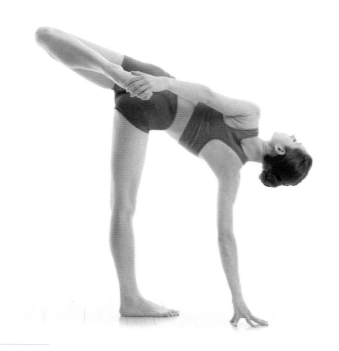

CHEST-OPENING TRICK

When opening the chest and shoulders in balance poses such as half moon and twisted half moon, it helps to keep your neck and chest relaxed. Easing up in the chest area allows you to rotate your torso more easily.

seated poses

Seated poses calm the body, release tension in the hips and hamstrings, and soothe the mind. They are used for warming up and cooling down, and for meditation.

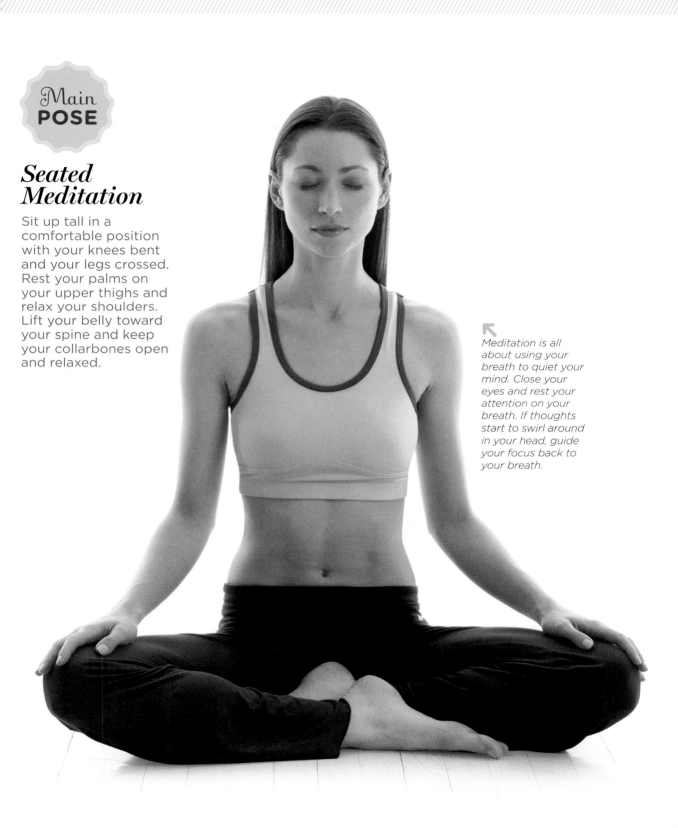

Seated Meditation

Sit up tall in a comfortable position with your knees bent and your legs crossed. Rest your palms on your upper thighs and relax your shoulders. Lift your belly toward your spine and keep your collarbones open and relaxed.

Meditation is all about using your breath to quiet your mind. Close your eyes and rest your attention on your breath. If thoughts start to swirl around in your head, guide your focus back to your breath.

Seated Meditation with Block

Sit on a block and fold your legs in so your knees relax out to the sides.

Using a block gives your hips and spine a chance to sit up straight without stressing your lower back.

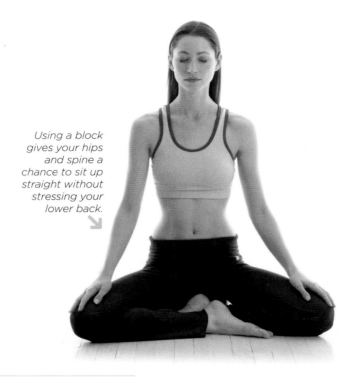

Seated Meditation, Arms in V

Sit up comfortably and lift your arms into a V shape. Use your inhales to lift some of the weight out of your body, and use your exhales to release tension. Relax your shoulders.

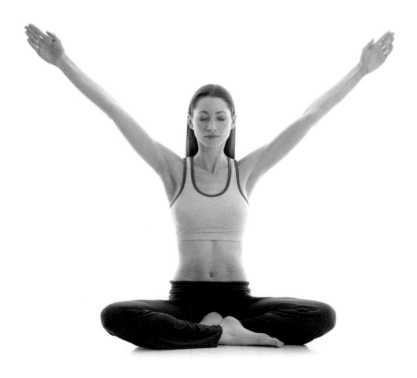

Seated Meditation, Arms Out to Sides

Sit up comfortably and extend your arms straight out to your sides, palms facing out.

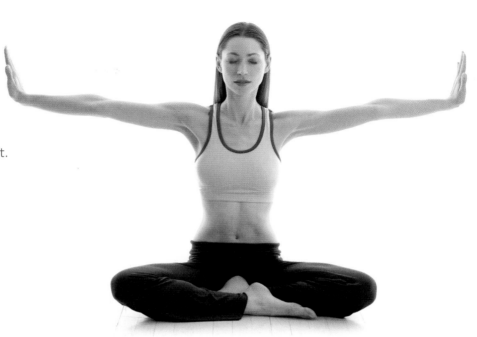

Seated Palm Press

Lace your fingers together and press your palms up toward the ceiling. Relax your shoulders so you have room around your neck, and look up at your hands. You can do this on a bed, couch, or chair with your legs uncrossed and your feet pressed firmly against the floor.

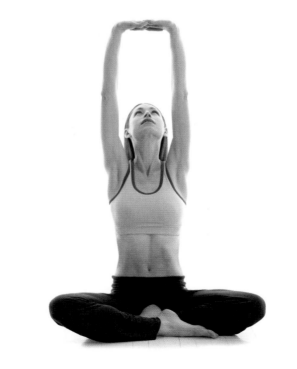

■ *Seated Side Release*

Stretch your right arm up and over your right ear. Bend from the waist to your left side and rest your left forearm on the floor. Turn your head to the right and look toward your right hand.

Breathe, and feel your ribs physically expand on the inhale and all the muscles release on the exhale.

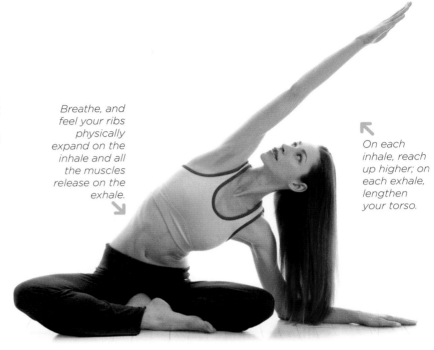

On each inhale, reach up higher; on each exhale, lengthen your torso.

■ *Seated Chest Opener*

Place the fingertips of both hands on the floor behind you. Press down with your fingertips and lift your chest up.

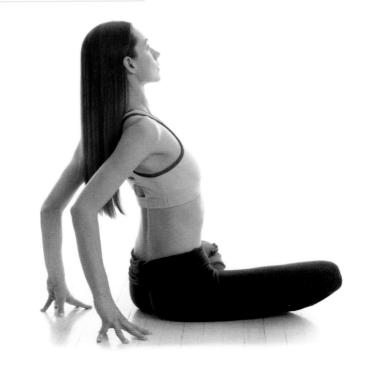

Seated Easy Twist

Bring your right hand to your left knee. Place the fingertips of your left hand on the floor behind you. Inhale and sit up tall. Exhale and twist around to the left.

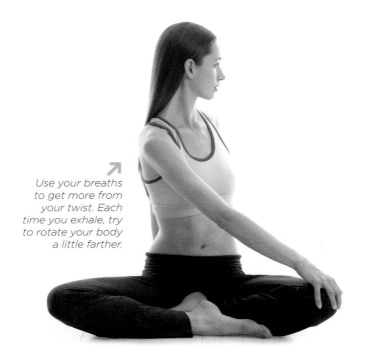

Use your breaths to get more from your twist. Each time you exhale, try to rotate your body a little farther.

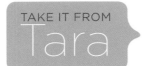

TAKE IT FROM
Tara

RELAX!

There is no extra credit in yoga for clenching muscles that you don't need for the movement. Unnecessary muscle engagement only inhibits building optimal strength and flexibility. Use what you need. Rest what you don't.

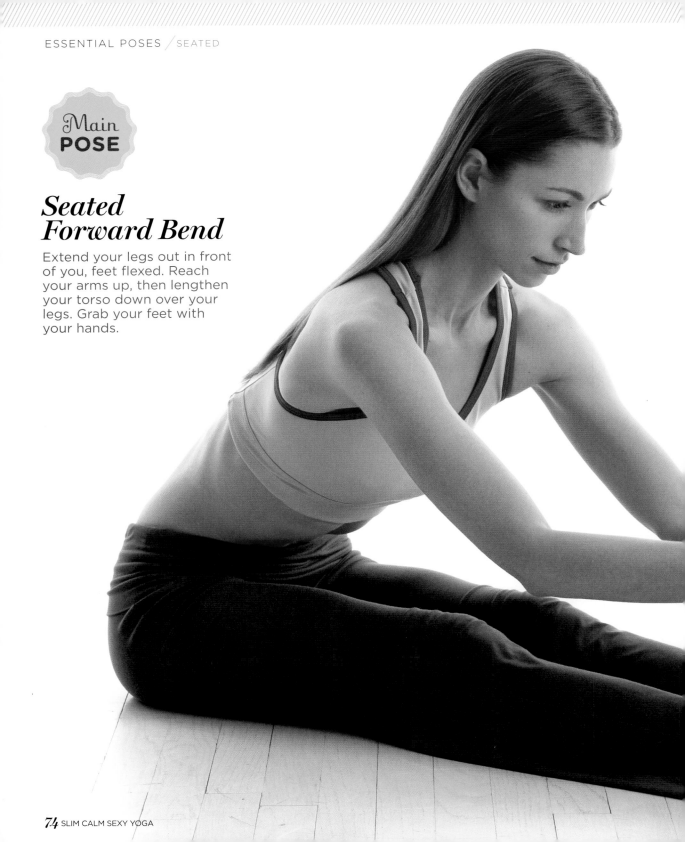

Main POSE

Seated Forward Bend

Extend your legs out in front of you, feet flexed. Reach your arms up, then lengthen your torso down over your legs. Grab your feet with your hands.

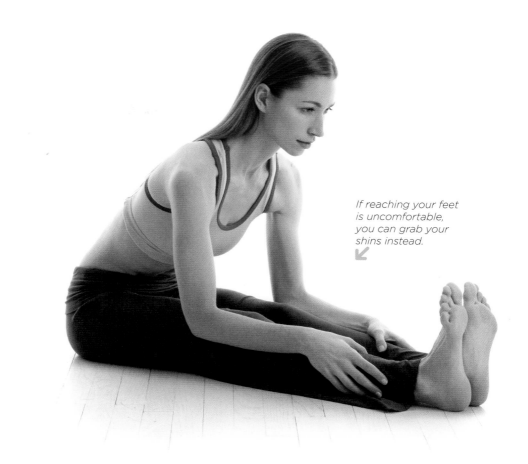

If reaching your feet is uncomfortable, you can grab your shins instead.

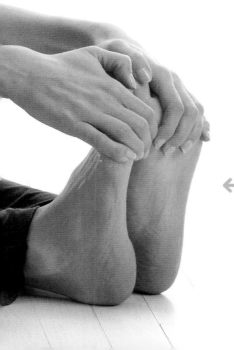

If your hamstrings or lower back are tight, bend your knees enough so you can rest your torso on your thighs. If you practice this way each day, you will start to notice your heels inching their way forward until one day you are in a forward bend with straight legs, your back long, and your torso resting on your legs.

■ *Seated Forward Bend, Bent Knees*

Bend your knees slightly. Flex your feet, reach your torso over your legs, and grab your toes. Relax your torso on your legs.

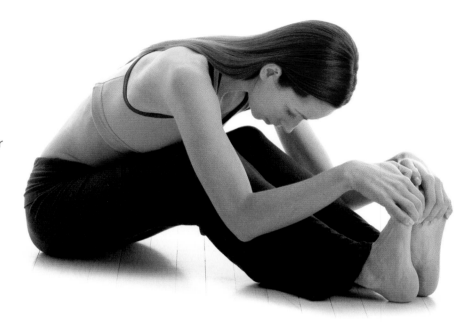

■ *Seated Forward Bend, Round Back*

Straighten your legs and round your back, looking down at your knees.

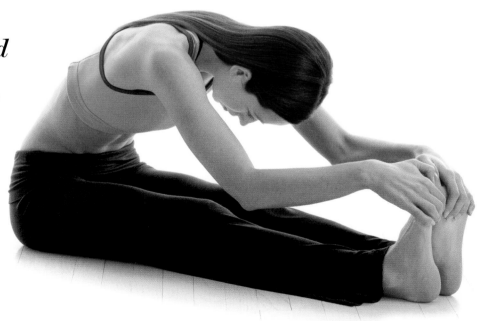

Seated Wide Leg Straddle

Extend your legs out to the sides, feet flexed. Bend forward at the hips and rest your forearms on the floor.

Use your breath to accomplish the most difficult movements, rather than relying on just your muscles. Each time you exhale, allow your legs to open up a bit more.

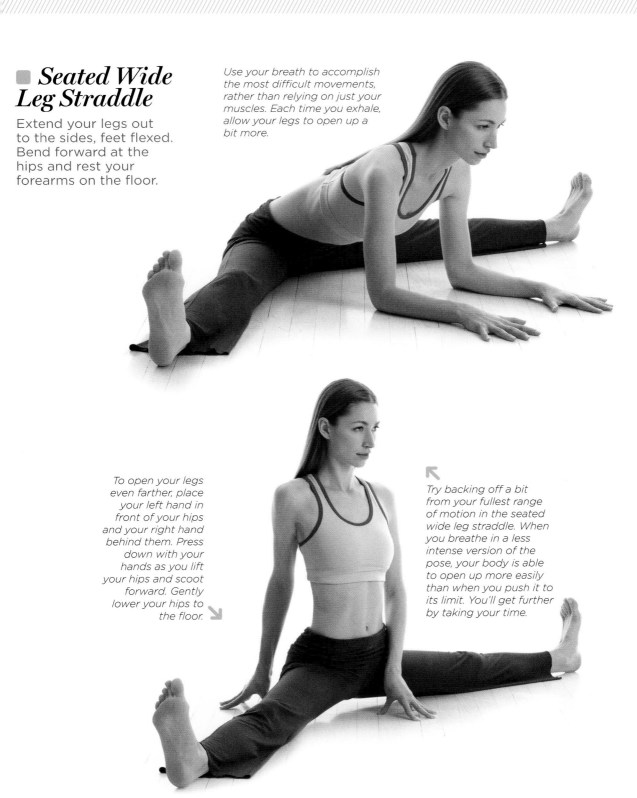

To open your legs even farther, place your left hand in front of your hips and your right hand behind them. Press down with your hands as you lift your hips and scoot forward. Gently lower your hips to the floor.

Try backing off a bit from your fullest range of motion in the seated wide leg straddle. When you breathe in a less intense version of the pose, your body is able to open up more easily than when you push it to its limit. You'll get further by taking your time.

■ Seated Wide Leg Straddle with Twist

Bring your left hand to your right foot and place the fingertips of your right hand on the floor beside you. Bend at the waist and extend your torso over your right leg. Look toward your right hand.

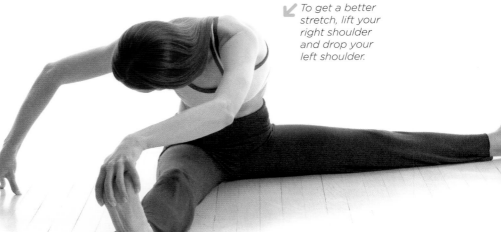

To get a better stretch, lift your right shoulder and drop your left shoulder.

■ Seated Open-Leg Forward Bend

Bring your legs in to the edges of your mat. Flex your feet and bend your knees slightly. Hold your feet with your hands, bend at your hips, and lengthen your torso over your legs.

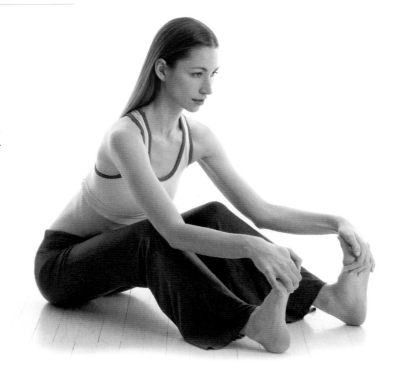

Seated Single-Leg Forward Bend

Bend your left knee and rest the bottom of your foot on your right inner thigh. Rest your left knee on the floor out to your left side. Reach your arms up overhead and inhale into your ribs. Exhale as you bring both hands to your right foot.

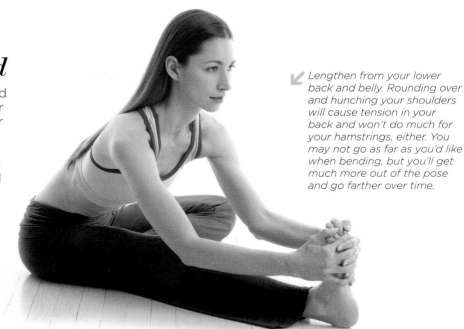

Lengthen from your lower back and belly. Rounding over and hunching your shoulders will cause tension in your back and won't do much for your hamstrings, either. You may not go as far as you'd like when bending, but you'll get much more out of the pose and go farther over time.

Seated Cross-Legged Easy Forward Bend

Cross your legs and gently bend forward at your hips, letting your hands stretch out straight in front of you on your mat. Breathe deeply and let all your muscles relax as you exhale.

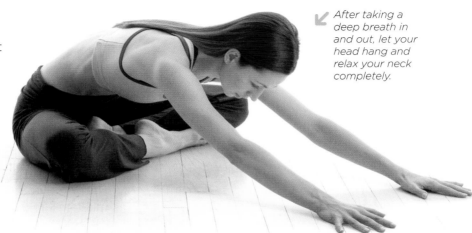

After taking a deep breath in and out, let your head hang and relax your neck completely.

■ *Seated Shin Hug*

Extend both legs forward and flex your feet. Bend your left knee, bringing your ankle in toward your hips. Bend your right knee and lift your right leg toward you so your shin is parallel to the floor. Bring the bottom of your right foot into your left elbow and wrap your right arm around your leg. Sit up tall as you move your leg closer to your chest.

TIP: *Try this with your hips on a blanket or block. Sitting with your hips higher than your knees allows extra room in your torso to extend straight up.*

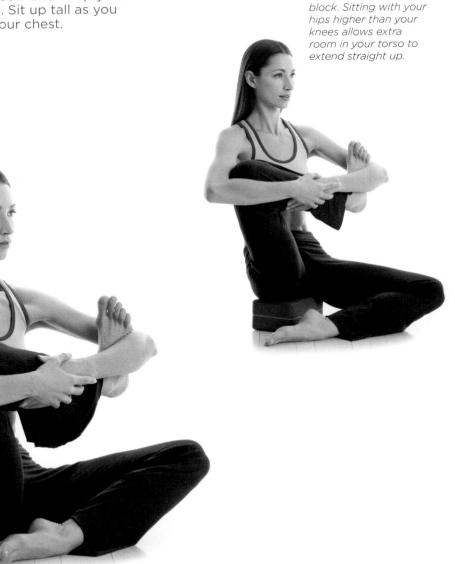

Seated Spine Twist

Extend your left leg and place your right foot on the outside of your left thigh. Inhale and extend your left arm straight up. As you exhale, wrap your left arm around your right knee. Press the fingertips of your right hand against the floor behind your hips.

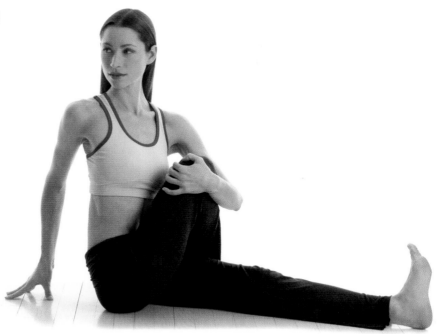

Think of your spine as a barbershop pole when you do a seated spine twist. Your torso is spiraling around your spine like the stripes on the pole. Inhale as you lift up tall. Exhale all the air out as you twist around farther. Repeat on each breath and you'll get the most out of your twist.

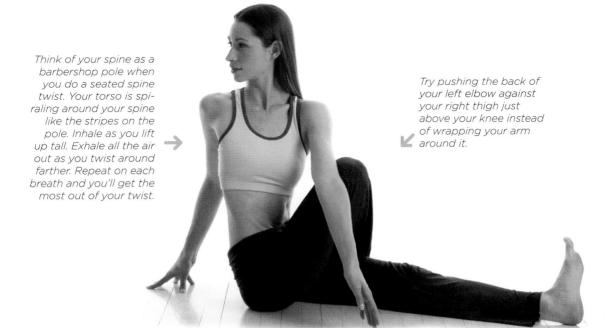

Try pushing the back of your left elbow against your right thigh just above your knee instead of wrapping your arm around it.

▪ *Bent Boat*

From a seated position,
legs extended in front
of you, bend your knees,
flex your feet, and raise
your shins until they're
parallel to the floor.
Place your arms outside
your shins, parallel to
the floor; lift your chest
and sit up tall.

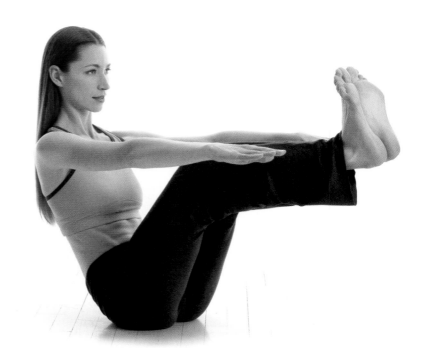

▪ *Boat Twist*

Dip your knees to one
side and bring your
arms to the other side.

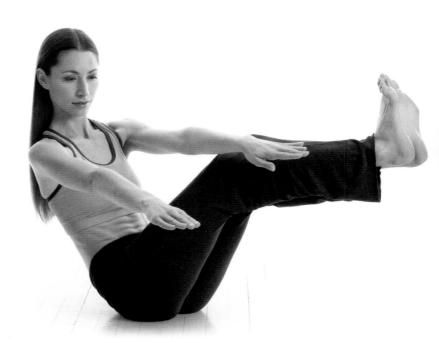

Spine Roll

Lie on your back. Bend your knees in and hug your shins. Gently rock forward and back on your spine. Start the movements small and gradually make them larger. Press each vertebra on the floor and treat this as a nice massage for your spine. Try to keep an equal distance between your head and your knees as you roll forward and back.

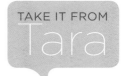

TAKE IT FROM Tara

CULTIVATE YOUR CORE

When doing any of these poses, lift your belly in and up. A common error in yoga and other physical activities is to push out your stomach during abdominal effort. Lifting your stomach in and up builds strength in the deeper layers of muscle and develops a strong core and flat stomach more efficiently than pushing out your belly on each crunch. Lifting in and up also helps with every other yoga pose, from down dog to handstands. When your core is strong, challenging poses become so much easier.

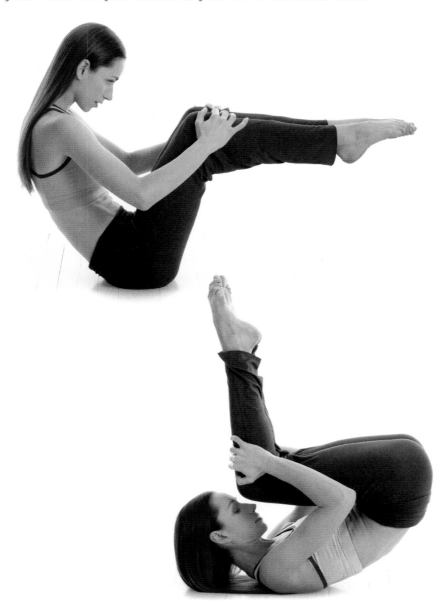

Three Wise Monkeys

The movements on these pages are borrowed from the Three Wise Monkeys maxim: See No Evil, Hear No Evil, and Speak No Evil. You may have seen statues of these three monkeys depicted together, one covering his eyes, one covering his ears, and one

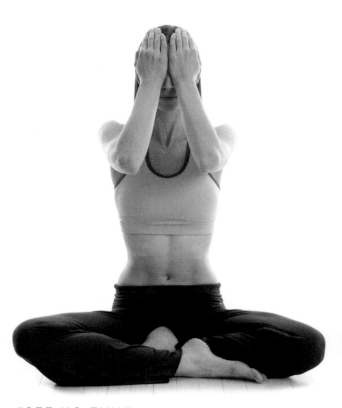

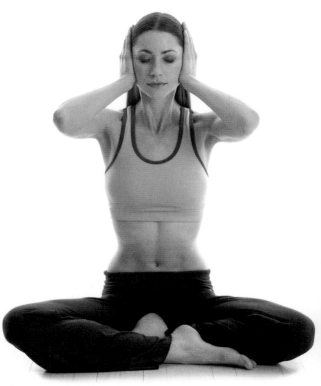

"SEE NO EVIL"
Eye Soother

Rub your palms together to create a little bit of heat in your hands. When your hands feel warm, close your eyes and place the heels of your hands gently over them. Let your fingers point upward and rest on your forehead.

This is great for eyestrain caused by too much computer-screen staring. It is also good for mild headaches and calming the brain.

"HEAR NO EVIL"
Ear Soother

Rub your palms together, creating heat, and place them over your ears. Let your fingers point upward and rest on the sides of your head.

This is great for silencing external noise. Just for a few moments, we come back to our breath and are shielded from outside distractions.

covering his mouth. Sometimes a fourth monkey is with them, crossing his arms. He is the Do No Evil monkey. The Three Wise Monkeys became popular from a 17th-century carving over a door of the famous Tōshō-gū shrine in Nikkō, Japan. The maxim probably came to Japan originally with a Tendai Buddhist legend from China in the 8th century. Our modern-day interpretation of the Three Wise Monkeys is intended to ward off anxiety, which can be interpreted as evil that is happening to the self.

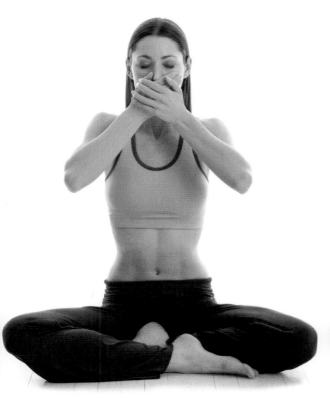

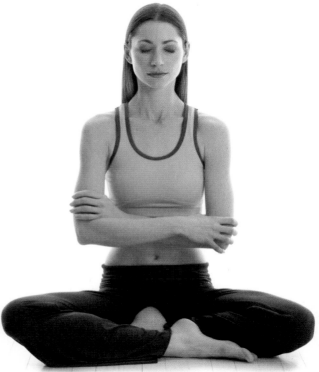

"SPEAK NO EVIL"

Jaw Soother

Rub your palms together and place your right hand over your mouth and your left hand on top of your right hand.

This is great for calming our impulses to speak without thinking.

"DO NO EVIL"

Crossed Arms

Cross your arms.

This is great for looking cool.

Main POSE

Hero

Sit on your heels and rest your palms in your lap. Rise up on your knees and separate your heels a little wider than your hips, keeping your knees as close together as you can. Gently move your calves to the sides with your thumbs, and lower your hips to the floor between your legs.

If you have any knee pain, sit on a block. →

Easy Hero Twist

Bring your left hand to your right knee and wrap your right hand around your back to grab your left hip. Gently squeeze your shoulder blades together, inhale, and sit up tall. Exhale and twist around to the right.

If you can't wrap your arm around your back, place the fingertips of your right hand on the floor behind you.

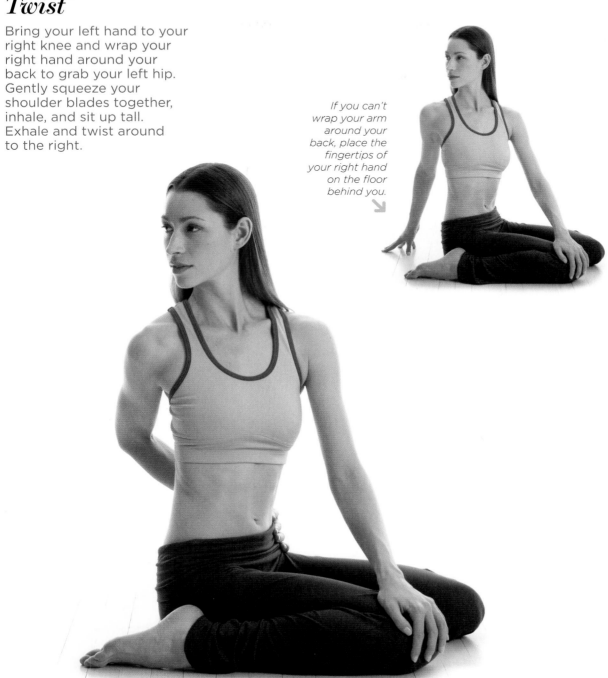

◼ *Cow Face*

Rise up on your knees. Cross your right leg in front of your left leg so your knees are touching and your right foot points to the left. Open your feet out to the sides. Gently ease your hips down. Rest your hands at your feet and relax your torso over your legs.

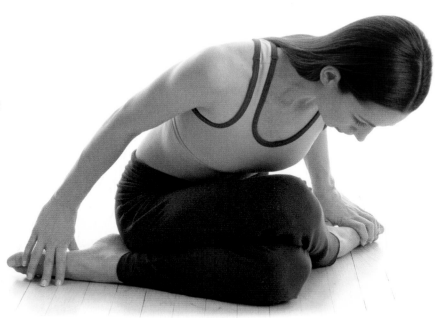

◼ *Ankle to Knee*

Place your right ankle on top of your left knee and open your hips so your right knee is on top of your left ankle.

You can help your hips open up in the ankle-to-knee pose by holding your right thigh and rotating it inward. This will help your hips release, and your knee will probably open up a bit more over your left ankle.

If your right knee is far from touching your left ankle, stay where you are and breathe.

If your knees and ankles meet, try walking your torso forward over your shins.

Compass Prep

Grab the outside of your left foot with your right hand. Cross your left arm over your left leg and rest your left hand on the floor near your right foot. Gently pull your left leg back until your left knee rests behind your left shoulder.

This is a great hip opener. →

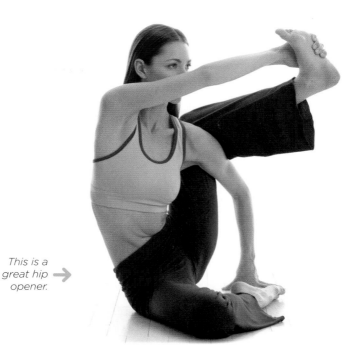

Compass

If you feel no tension in compass prep, straighten your left leg as you open your shoulders and lean your spine on your left leg. Look up under your right arm.

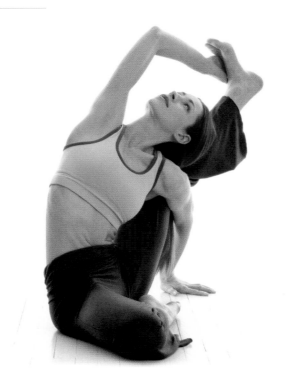

Pigeon

Sit on your heels, then move your right foot in front of you and over to the left side of your mat, and ease your right knee down toward the right side of your mat. Your right shin should be as parallel as you can get it to the front of your mat. Extend your left leg behind you. Walk your hands forward over your right leg. If you can, rest your forehead on the floor.

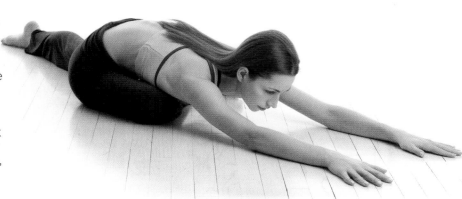

Split with Block under Hip

Grab a block and position it under your right hip. Flex your right foot and extend your right leg forward on your mat. Extend your left leg behind you. Keep your hips square by pulling your right hip back and into the socket and guiding your left hip forward.

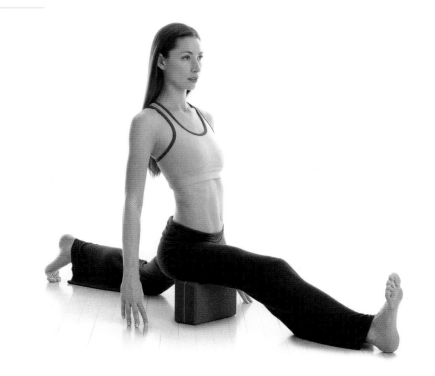

Split with Two Blocks

Grab a block in each hand and press the blocks down on the mat at your sides, next to your hips. Lift your torso and extend your right leg forward on your mat. Extend your left leg behind you. Keep your hips square by pulling your right hip back and into the socket and guiding your left hip forward.

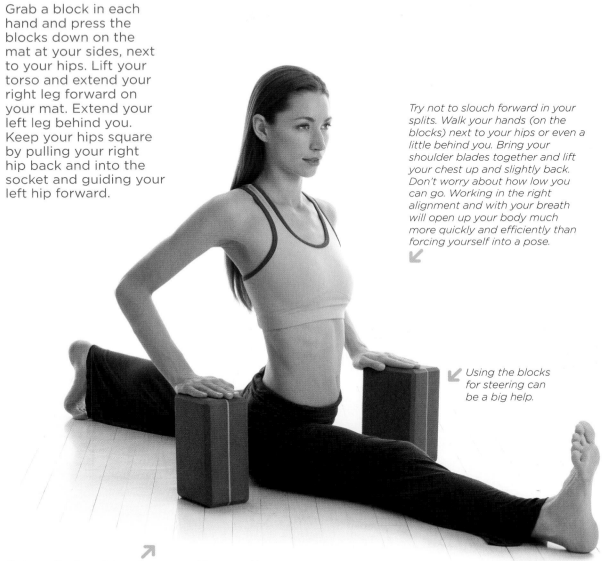

Try not to slouch forward in your splits. Walk your hands (on the blocks) next to your hips or even a little behind you. Bring your shoulder blades together and lift your chest up and slightly back. Don't worry about how low you can go. Working in the right alignment and with your breath will open up your body much more quickly and efficiently than forcing yourself into a pose.

Using the blocks for steering can be a big help.

Doing splits doesn't have to mean getting your hips on the floor and raising your arms like a gymnast. When you use blocks to prop yourself up, you can stay and breathe into the tension in manageable increments. With time and patience, your hamstrings and hips will open up. Keep practicing.

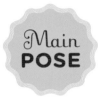

Main
POSE

Child's Pose

Kneel and sit back on your heels.
Extend your torso over your legs
and rest your forehead on the floor.
Relax your neck and shoulders.

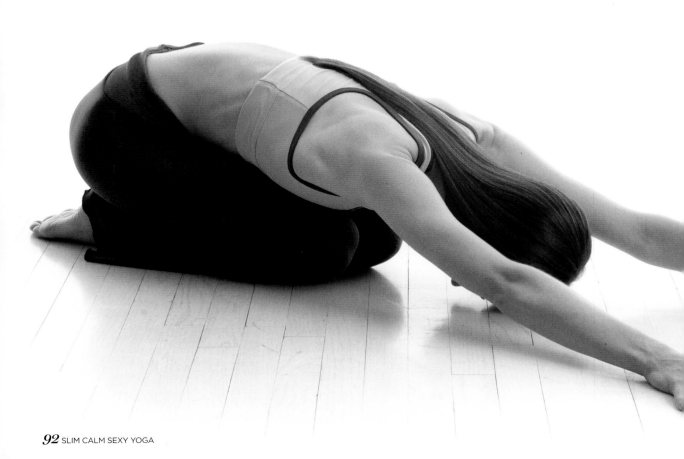

Child's Pose Twist

Thread your left arm under your right arm and rest your left shoulder and ear on the floor. If your hips have lifted, gently lower them back toward your heels.

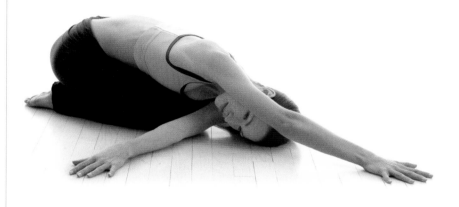

Sit on Heels

Sit up straight and rest your palms on your thighs.

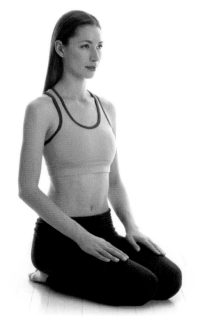

arm balances & inversions

ARM BALANCES
Balancing on your arms
strengthens and tones the entire body while targeting the abdominals, shoulders, and arms. Working on arm balances builds focus in the mind and enhances total body coordination and awareness. These poses are commonly used to build heat in the body.

Plank

Come to your hands and knees. Tuck your toes under and straighten your legs so you are in one horizontal line.

Extend forward through the top of your head and reach back through your heels. Reach the backs of your legs up.

Bring your shoulder blades together.

Keep your elbows straight but not locked. Working with locked elbows is like slouching. You might be able to hold the position more easily, but it won't help you build strength because you rely on the joint to do the work instead of relying on your muscles. Back off slightly from your hyperextended position so your elbows are straight. In plank, your elbows should be facing back toward your feet. Working this way will build strong and sexy shoulders.

Make sure your hands are under your shoulders and your fingers are spread wide, as if you were squishing them into wet sand. Spreading your fingers ensures a stable foundation that builds strength effectively and prevents injury.

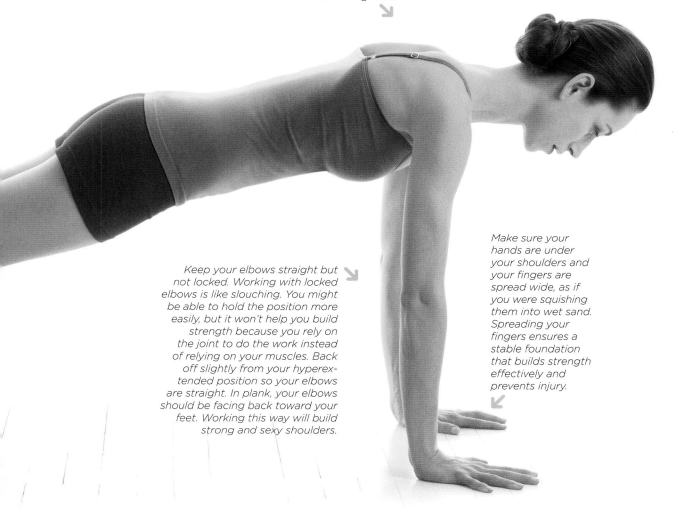

Half Pushup

Bend your elbows so they point straight back along your ribs and lower yourself halfway to the floor. Pause when your upper arms are parallel to the floor.

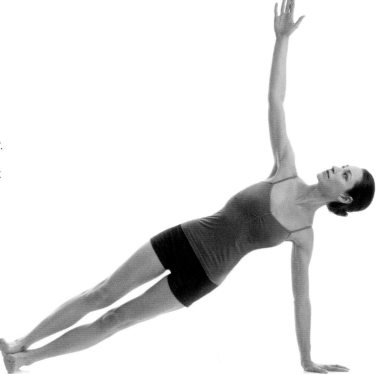

Reach out forward through the top of your head and back through your heels.

Lift your stomach up and in to keep your body in one straight line.

Side Plank

Press your left hand firmly against the floor and roll to the outside edge of your left foot, stacking your right ankle, hip, and shoulder on top of your left ankle, hip, and shoulder. Reach straight up with your right arm and look up toward your hand.

Plank Forearm

Get into a plank pose resting
on your forearms.

*Extend forward
through the top
of your head and
reach back through
your heels.*

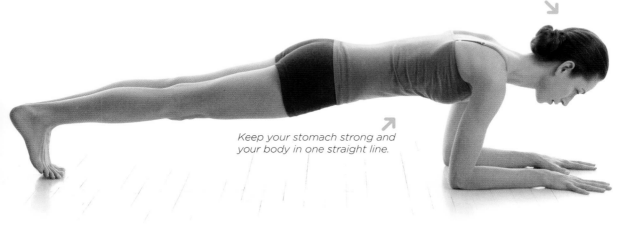

*Keep your stomach strong and
your body in one straight line.*

Plank Split

Lift your left leg
and bring your body
forward so your shoul-
ders stack on top of
your wrists.

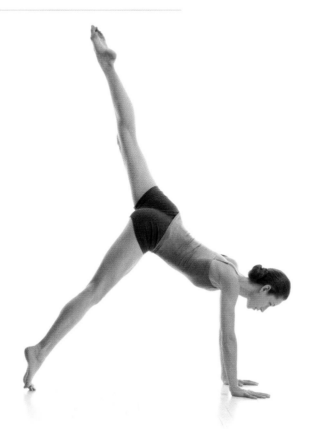

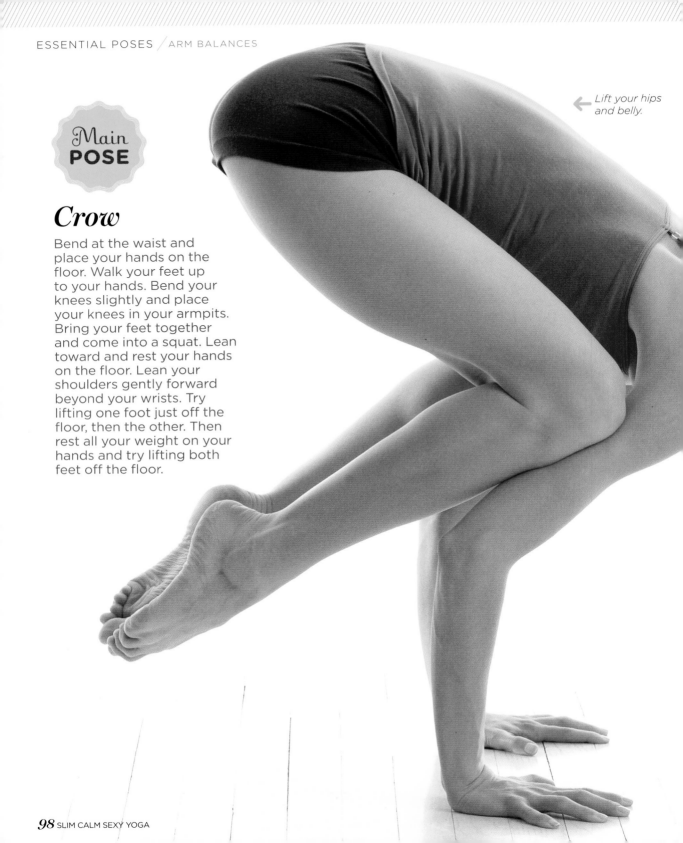

Lift your hips and belly.

Main POSE

Crow

Bend at the waist and place your hands on the floor. Walk your feet up to your hands. Bend your knees slightly and place your knees in your armpits. Bring your feet together and come into a squat. Lean toward and rest your hands on the floor. Lean your shoulders gently forward beyond your wrists. Try lifting one foot just off the floor, then the other. Then rest all your weight on your hands and try lifting both feet off the floor.

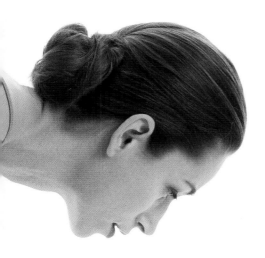

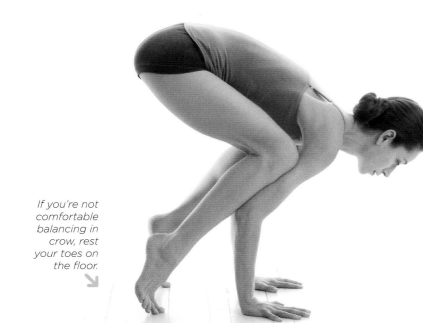

If you're not comfortable balancing in crow, rest your toes on the floor.

TAKE IT FROM
Tara

BE WHERE YOU ARE

If you are unable to lift your feet off the floor in crow pose, that's completely fine. You'll build strength by pressing the floor away and lifting up in your hips and stomach. Eventually, with practice, you will be able to come into crow, and when you do, you'll find yet another pose to master. There will always be another pose learn, so don't worry about it and just be present where you are.

■ *Side Crow*

Bring your toes back to the floor, then swivel your knees to the right. Press your left thigh on the back of your right upper arm. Lean your shoulders out past your thighs and carefully try lifting your toes off the floor.

If you have trouble balancing in side crow, let your feet rest on the floor. ↘

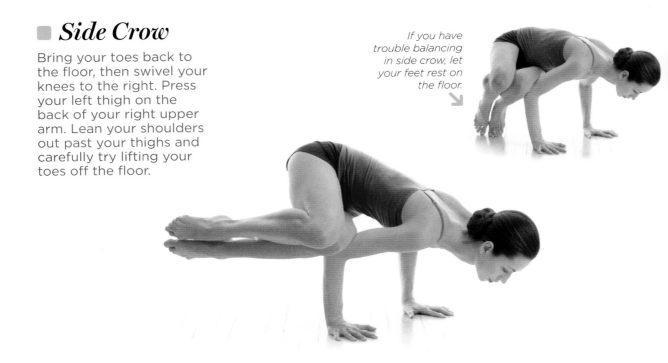

■ *Half Crow Lift*

From crow, lift your hips and bring your right knee to the outside of your right shoulder.

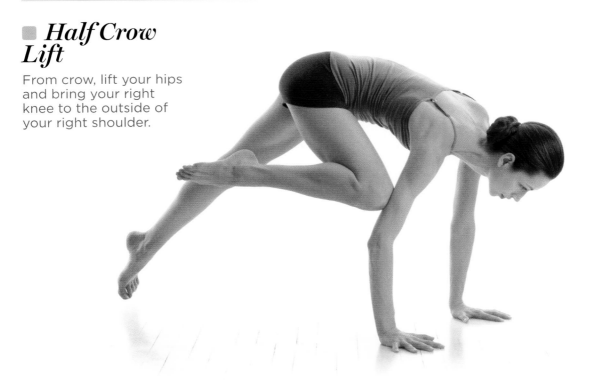

Knee to Forehead

Lift your hips and bring your right knee to your forehead. Roll your upper back forward.

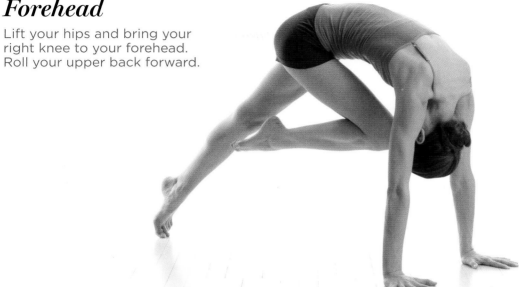

Knee Cross Lift

Bend your elbows and bring your right knee across to the back of your left upper arm. Roll onto the inner edges of the toes of your left foot.

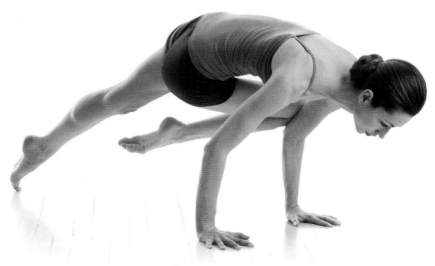

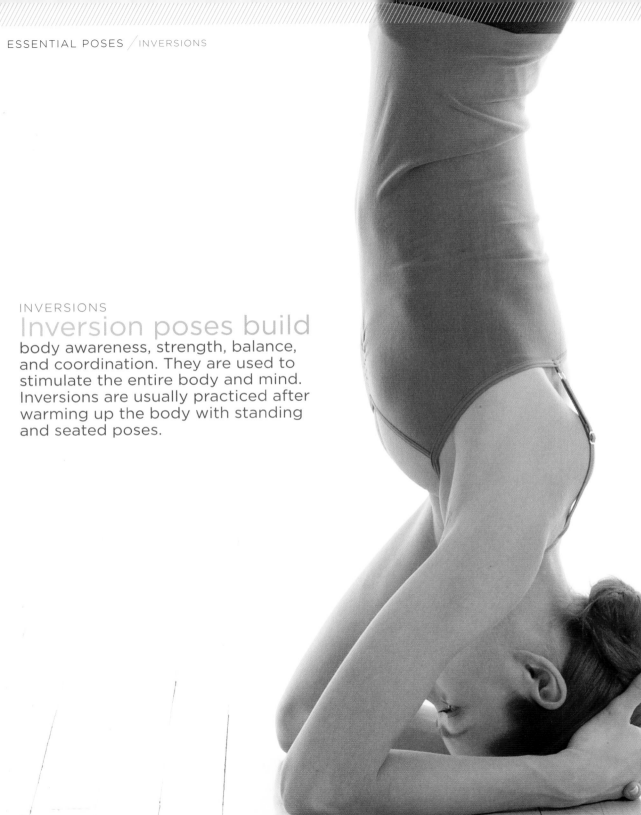

INVERSIONS
Inversion poses build
body awareness, strength, balance, and coordination. They are used to stimulate the entire body and mind. Inversions are usually practiced after warming up the body with standing and seated poses.

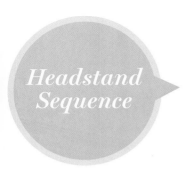

Headstand Sequence

Proper alignment is everything in a headstand. You can't fake it with this one. Practice the moves that strengthen and open you until you can get your hips directly above your shoulders. Once you're comfortable and have your alignment down, you can start to move into a full headstand. Give your full attention to all the steps along the way—it's hard work, but you'll be rewarded for not rushing.

■ *Headstand Sock Slide*

Put on a pair of socks. I know, unusual for yoga, but this is a fun one that builds strength, too!

Kneel on the floor facing your mat. Lace your fingers together and place your forearms on the floor, keeping your elbows shoulder-width apart. Place the top of your head on the mat so the palms of your hands are cradling the back of your head. Tuck your toes under and straighten your legs **[A]**. Engage your abs, pulling your belly in, and slide your feet toward your head until your hips are above your shoulders **[B]**.

TIP: *Even if you are brand new to headstand, this position is a nonscary introduction. Make sure the very top of your head is on the floor. Often when people are new to headstand, they place their foreheads or the backs of their heads on the floor.*

TIP: *Fold your yoga mat in half to make it a little thicker for your head. You can also use a rug for this one.*

TIP: *This movement strengthens your core and works toward getting your hips on top of your shoulders. This helps with the alignment, strength, and balance you will need for a full headstand.*

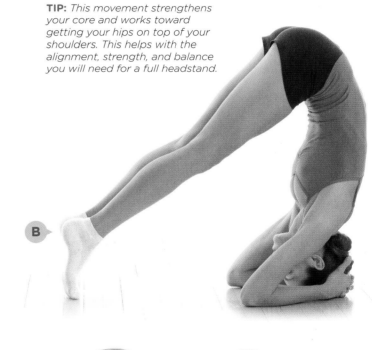

■ *Headstand Prep, Feet Walked In*

Take off your socks. Come back into the initial sock slide position. Walk your feet in a couple of inches and stay there for 5 breaths. Walk your feet in a couple more inches and stay there for 5 breaths. Repeat until your hips are directly on top of your shoulders.

■ *Headstand Prep, One Heel to Hip*

From the position in which your hips are directly above your shoulders, carefully bend your left knee, bringing your left heel toward your hip. Stay here for 5 breaths and lower your foot back down to the floor. Try the other heel.

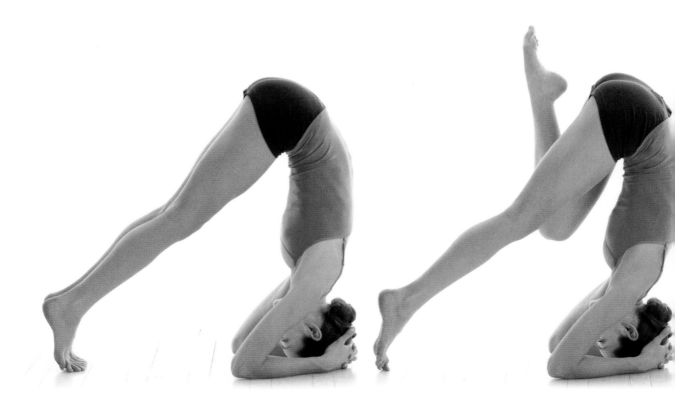

Headstand Prep, Both Heels to Hips

After you're comfortable bringing each heel to your hip separately and holding it there, try bringing both heels to your hips. Stay here for 5 breaths and slowly lower both feet back down to the floor.

Headstand Prep Leg Lift, Square Hips

After you're comfortable bringing both heels to your hips, try extending your right leg straight out, parallel to the floor, keeping the toes of your left foot on the floor. Keep your hips square. Stay here for 5 breaths. Lower your right leg and try it with your left. Hold for 5 breaths, then lower your left leg. Try it with both legs.

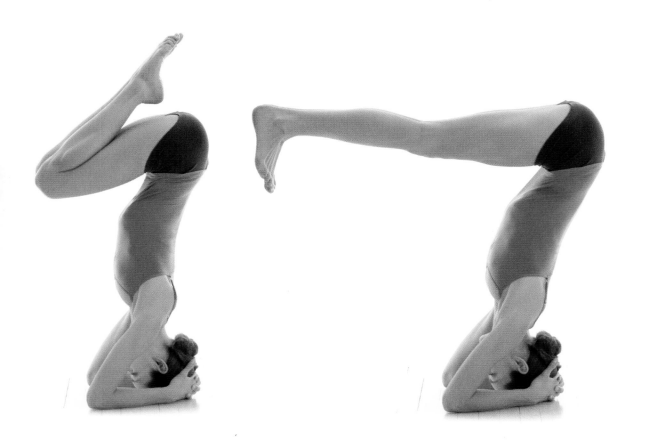

Headstand

After you're comfortable with the previous headstand prep poses, walk your feet in until your hips are stacked on top of your shoulders. Bring one heel to your hip and then the other. Carefully and slowly lift and straighten your legs. Lower yourself the same way you came up.

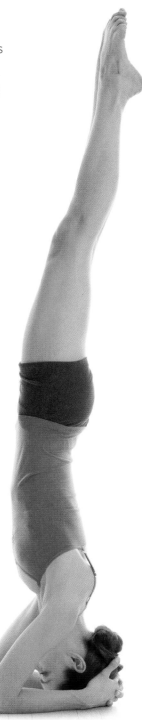

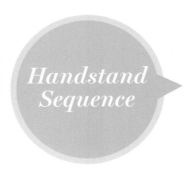

Proper alignment makes or breaks a handstand. Your ability to balance may change from day to day, so try not to have expectations when you practice. Instead, keep your focus and you will nail it more often than not. When you are focused and take your time working through all the steps that lead up to the full pose, you'll build strength and remain comfortable enough to keep breathing easily, and soon enough you'll be sticking your handstands consistently.

Forearm Stand Prep

From down dog, bend your elbows and lower your forearms to the floor.

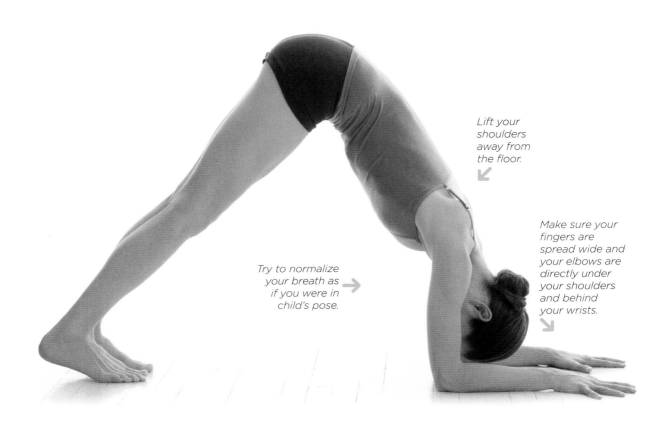

Lift your shoulders away from the floor.

Try to normalize your breath as if you were in child's pose.

Make sure your fingers are spread wide and your elbows are directly under your shoulders and behind your wrists.

Forearm Stand Leg Raise

Walk your feet in about 6 inches, moving your hips over your shoulders. Inhale and lift your left leg, bringing your hips higher over your shoulders. Try to roll onto the toes of your right foot.

Forearm Stand

When you're comfortable raising one leg, try raising both.

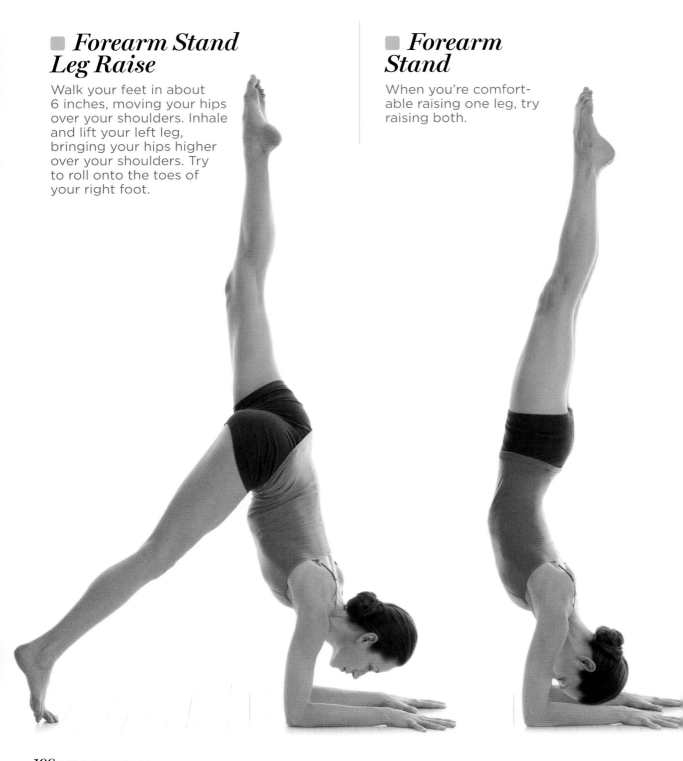

Handstand at Wall

Place your hands on the floor about a foot away from a wall. Press to a down dog. Walk your feet in and extend your right leg straight up. Rock up with your leg straight, bringing your right foot to the wall and following immediately with your left, bringing it to rest against the wall, too. You can play with balance here by moving one leg at a time away from the wall.

TIP: *It's good to try handstands in the middle of the room so you don't become dependent on a wall, but it is also occasionally useful to practice using the wall. Staying in handstand at the wall also helps you build the strength in your arms and core that you'll need to hold the position on your own.*

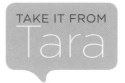
ONE STEP AT A TIME

There's no need to launch yourself into a position if your body isn't ready to go there. There are no shortcuts with yoga. Something good to consider: Any given pose includes everything that comes before it as well as everything that follows it. By those standards, if you launch into what looks like the pose, you're not really doing the pose.

Jumping into a position can also cause injury. Even if you remain injury-free, training your body to move into something when it's not ready is a bad habit that works against building strength and focus. When you leap rather than move easily from a steady base, you train your mind to be dissatisfied with where you are. Practice working where you are.

■ *Handstand*

Come into down dog. Walk your feet about a foot closer to your hands. Raise one leg up high and keep your hips square. Press your palms down firmly **[A]**. Bend your leg, rock your shoulders ahead of your wrists and your hips over your shoulders, and raise it off the floor **[B]**. When you find a balance, draw your legs slowly together until they both extend straight up **[C]**.

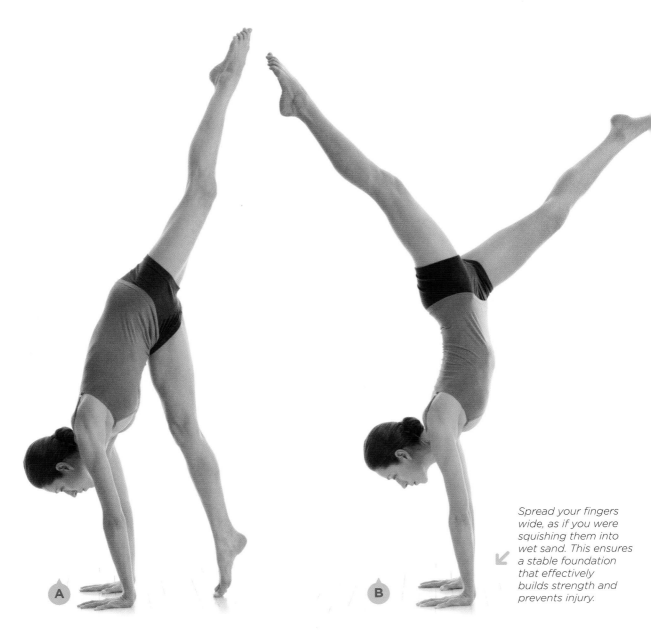

Spread your fingers wide, as if you were squishing them into wet sand. This ensures a stable foundation that effectively builds strength and prevents injury.

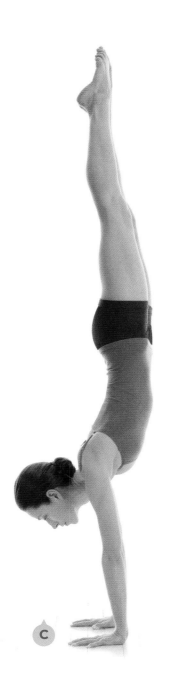

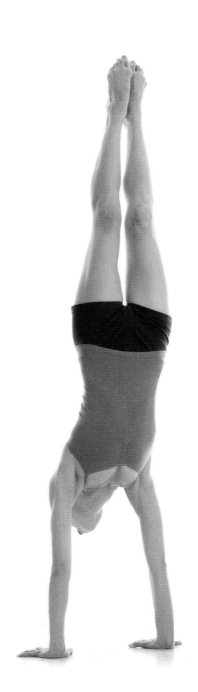

TAKE IT FROM
Tara

PRACTICE
SAFELY!

Learning a hand-stand comes with a lot of falling. Move any furniture with hard edges out of the way, and try to practice on a mat or soft carpeting. Remember to have fun, and don't take yourself too seriously. Spontaneous laughter is good!

C

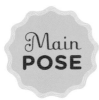

Main POSE

Plow

Lie flat on your back and extend your legs straight up above your hips. Flex your feet, press your arms along your sides, and gently peel your spine off the floor, reaching your legs straight behind you until your toes find the floor. Gently press into the balls of your feet and reach your heels toward the floor.

If your feet don't touch the floor, stay where you feel a little bit of tension and try to use your breath to gently lower your feet little by little on each exhale. If you feel any neck or back discomfort, don't try to push to make your feet reach the floor.

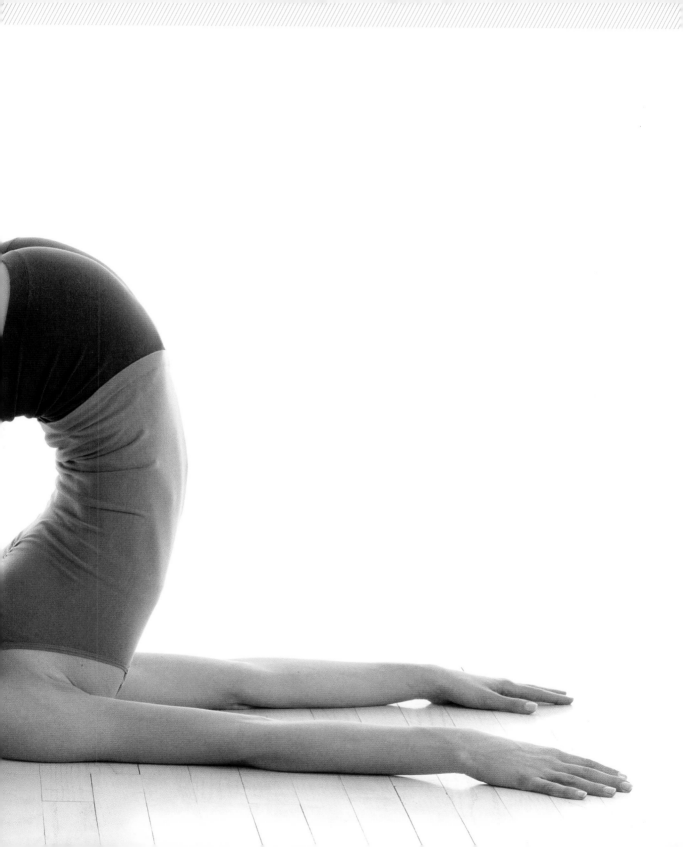

■ *Shoulder Stand*

Press your hands against your middle back. Work your hands along your spine toward your shoulders. When you feel steady, gently reach your legs up toward vertical. Stay here for 30 long, deep breaths. To come out of the pose, slowly lower yourself back to plow. Bend your knees slightly and roll down vertebra by vertebra until you're lying flat on your back.

TIP: *If your feet are far from reaching the floor in plow and you feel tension in your back, stay in plow and breathe. Try a shoulder stand only if your feet touch the floor in plow and your neck and spine feel okay.*

■ *Legs up the Wall*

Sit with your legs stretched out in front of you and your side right next to a wall. Lie down, bring your torso perpendicular to the wall, and walk your legs up the wall. Keep your legs straight and feet flexed. Rest your arms on your abdomen or by your sides on the mat.

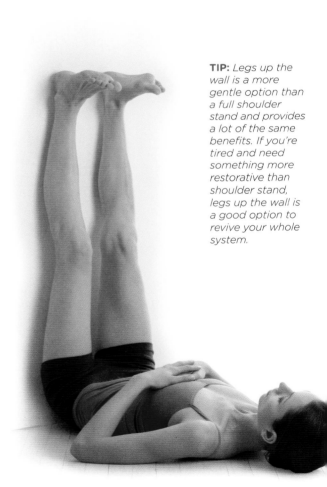

TIP: *Legs up the wall is a more gentle option than a full shoulder stand and provides a lot of the same benefits. If you're tired and need something more restorative than shoulder stand, legs up the wall is a good option to revive your whole system.*

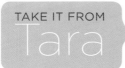

TAKE IT FROM
Tara

IT'S NOT ABOUT DOING THE POSE PERFECTLY!

Yoga is more about soaking up the benefits of the poses than performing impressive positions. And the poses are designed to stimulate, energize, and rejuvenate your system.

other poses

Lying-Down Poses, Back Bends, and Partner-Supported Poses

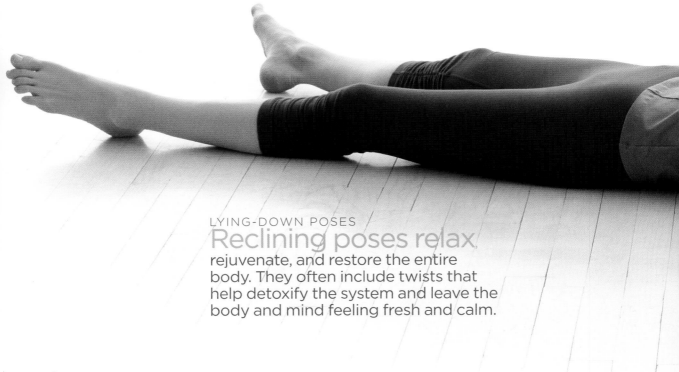

LYING-DOWN POSES
Reclining poses relax,
rejuvenate, and restore the entire body. They often include twists that help detoxify the system and leave the body and mind feeling fresh and calm.

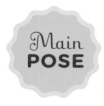

Lying-Down V

Lie on your back, stretch your
arms out on the floor over your
head in a V, and extend your legs
slightly wider than your hips.

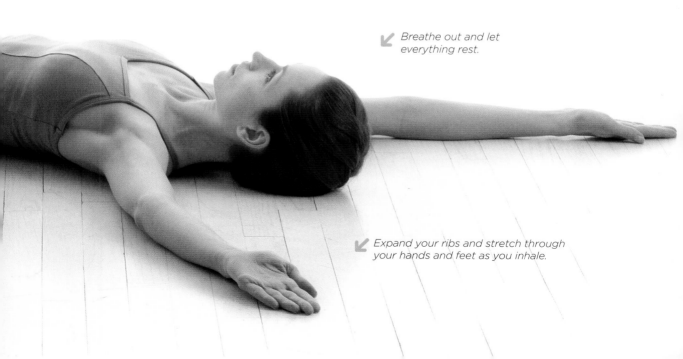

*Breathe out and let
everything rest.*

*Expand your ribs and stretch through
your hands and feet as you inhale.*

■ *V Twist*

Reach your right leg across your left leg and rest your right foot on the floor. Let your right arm come off the floor and extend out through your right fingertips. Direct your gaze to the right side.

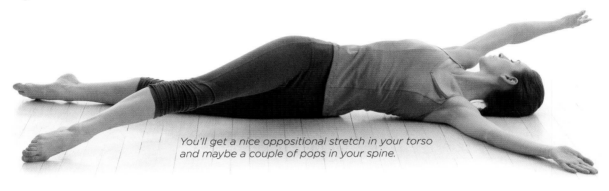

Breathe deeply and use your exhales to relax further into the twist.

You'll get a nice oppositional stretch in your torso and maybe a couple of pops in your spine.

■ *Knee-to-Chest Circle*

Gently bring your right knee to your chest and hold your shin with both hands. Carefully move your knee around in little circles to the left for a few breaths, and then to the right.

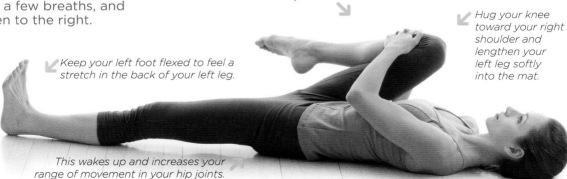

You can place your left hand on the front of your left thigh to make sure your hip is nice and relaxed.

Hug your knee toward your right shoulder and lengthen your left leg softly into the mat.

Keep your left foot flexed to feel a stretch in the back of your left leg.

This wakes up and increases your range of movement in your hip joints.

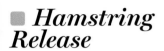 ## *Hamstring Release*

Straighten your right leg and hold your right calf with both hands. Extend your left leg, raising your left foot and your head and shoulders off the floor. Point your toes and relax your shoulders.

Half Happy Baby

Bend your right knee and flex your foot to face the ceiling. Grab the outside of your right foot with your right hand and bend your knee toward your armpit. Point the toes of your left foot.

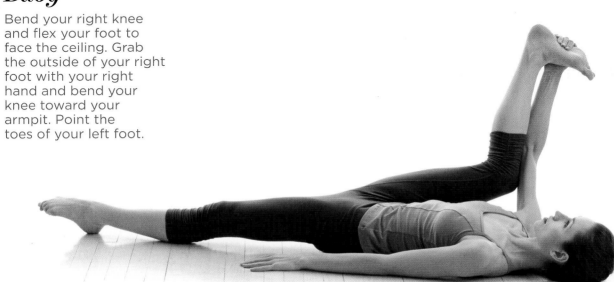

Happy Baby

Bend both knees and flex your feet to face the ceiling. Grab the outside of each foot with your hands and bend your knees toward your armpits.

Knee Cross

Lace your fingers together behind your head. Bend your left knee in to your chest and bring your right elbow across your body and to the outside of your knee.

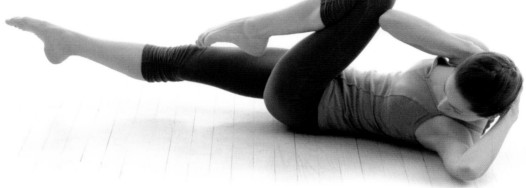

Knee Hug

Hug both knees to your chest and rock slowly from side to side on your back. Breathe deeply and slowly. Let your whole back relax into your mat.

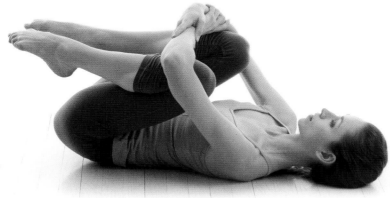

Reclining Goddess

Bring the soles of your feet together and let your knees relax out to the sides. Extend your arms out to the sides. Bend your elbows at right angles so your hands point above your head.

Relax your shoulders and hips into the floor on each exhale.

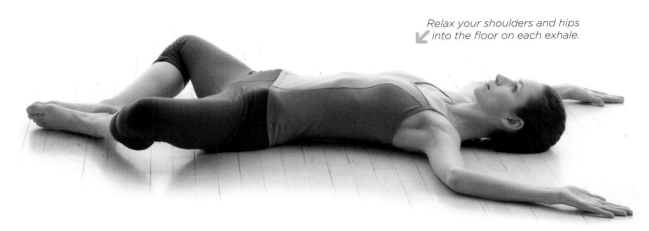

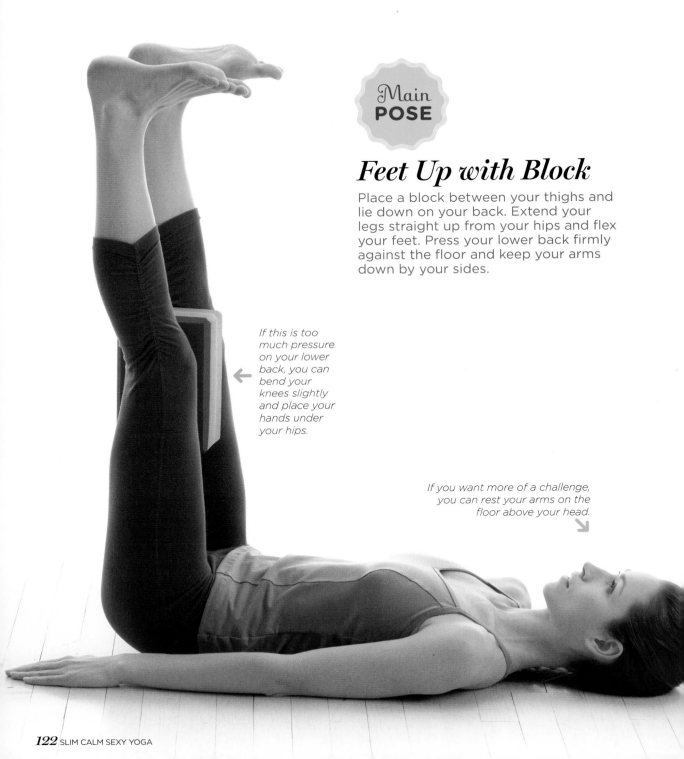

Main POSE

Feet Up with Block

Place a block between your thighs and lie down on your back. Extend your legs straight up from your hips and flex your feet. Press your lower back firmly against the floor and keep your arms down by your sides.

If this is too much pressure on your lower back, you can bend your knees slightly and place your hands under your hips.

If you want more of a challenge, you can rest your arms on the floor above your head.

Leg Raise with Block

With straight legs, lower your heels toward the floor as much as you can while keeping your lower back against the floor. Pause at the low point and then lift your legs back up to vertical.

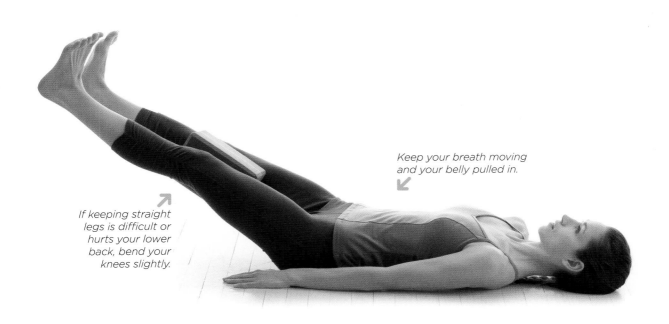

Keep your breath moving and your belly pulled in.

If keeping straight legs is difficult or hurts your lower back, bend your knees slightly.

■ *Hover with Block*

Lie down and extend your legs straight out with your toes pointed. Keep your feet, head, and shoulders raised off the floor and reach your arms straight out toward your knees. Press your lower back against the floor.

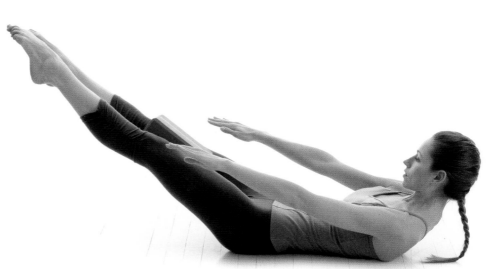

■ *Knee to Chest*

Bring your right knee to your chest and wrap your hands or arms around your shin to pull it gently closer to you.

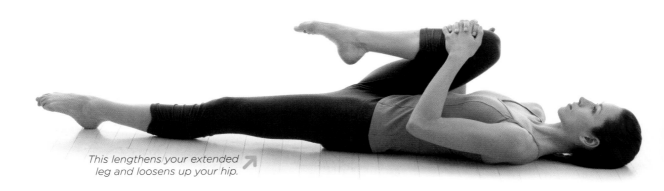

This lengthens your extended leg and loosens up your hip.

Single Leg Extension

Extend your right leg straight up toward the ceiling, foot flexed. Hold your leg with both hands behind your knee or closer to your ankle. Keep your leg straight and bring it closer to your head on each exhale. Lower it slowly.

Remember to stay gentle with these stretches so they are more of a release than a stretch.

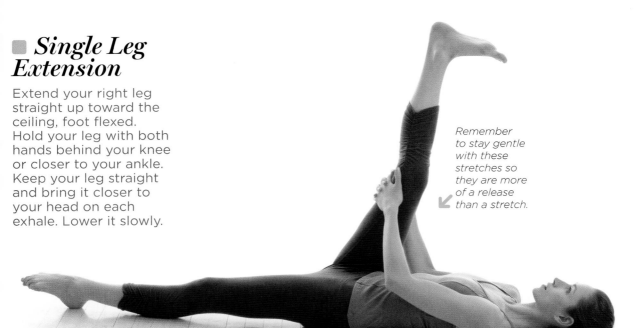

Spine Twist

Bring your right knee to your chest and twist it across your body until your right knee rests on the floor. Turn your head to the right and bring your arms out so your upper body forms a T shape.

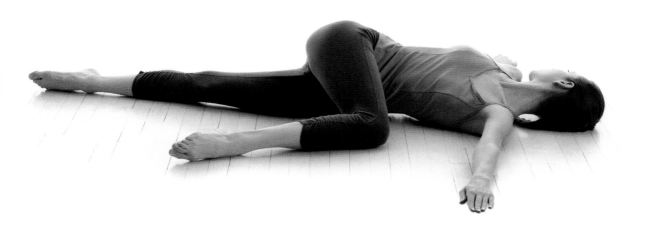

■ *Hip Release, Foot in Elbow*

Place the bottom of your right foot in the crook of your left elbow. Let your right knee fall out to the right side, and wrap your arms around your leg. Inhale and lengthen your spine. Exhale and draw your leg closer to you.

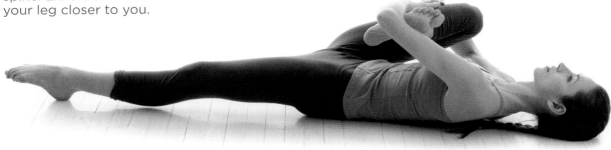

■ *Corpse*

Lie with both legs straight and resting on the floor in front of you. Relax your arms by your sides. Close your eyes and breathe deeply into your belly to release any leftover tension. Let your breathing return to normal and rest here.

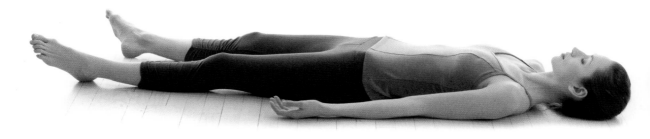

Supported Corpse with Blocks

Place a block lengthwise on your mat. Lie on your back with the block between your shoulder blades and rest your spine along the block, keeping your hips on the floor. Put a second block vertically under your head.

Propping yourself up on blocks helps to open your chest, spine, and hips.

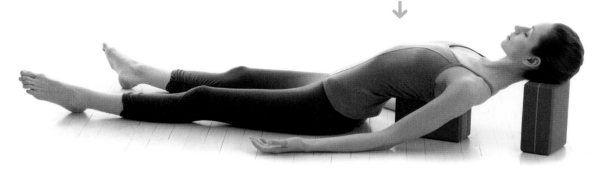

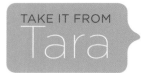
CLEAR YOUR MIND

The point of corpse pose is to practice doing nothing. This can be very difficult, but it's an important part of letting your body soak in all the benefits of your work. If your attention strays off to thinking, try returning your focus to breathing and relaxing your whole body, as well as your mind.

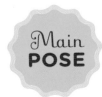

Main
POSE

Cat

Come to all fours. Spread your fingers wide and make sure your hands are under your shoulders and your knees are under your hips. Inhale, tuck your tailbone, round your back, and look toward your belly.

BACK BENDS

Back bends strengthen and
lengthen the entire spine and open the hips. They help improve posture, relieve tension in tight shoulders, and ease mild back pain. Simple back bends can be used to warm up the body, and deeper back bends are best done after the body has been warmed up with some standing and seated poses.

Back bending is more about opening and releasing tension than about pushing to get yourself into a pose. You may need to spend time using blocks and breathing deeply to release tension in tight areas to do some of these poses. Forcing and pushing isn't a great idea in any pose, but it simply won't work when it comes to back bends. Yoga creates a balance of strength and flexibility. You need both to be really strong. Too much muscular strength without flexibility restricts movement. Too much flexibility without strength in the muscles creates instability. Both imbalances can lead to injury and roadblocks.

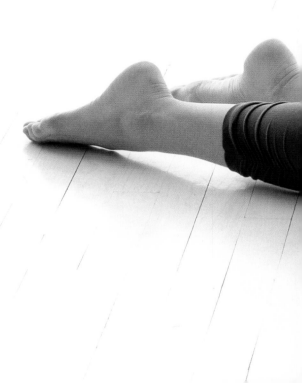

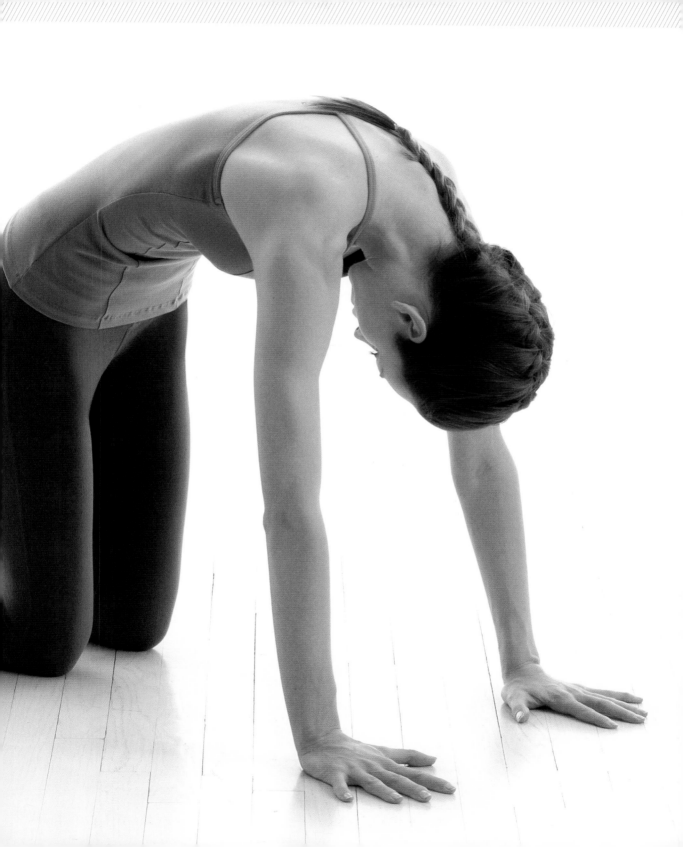

▪ *Cow*

Exhale, drop your belly,
arch your lower back,
and look up.

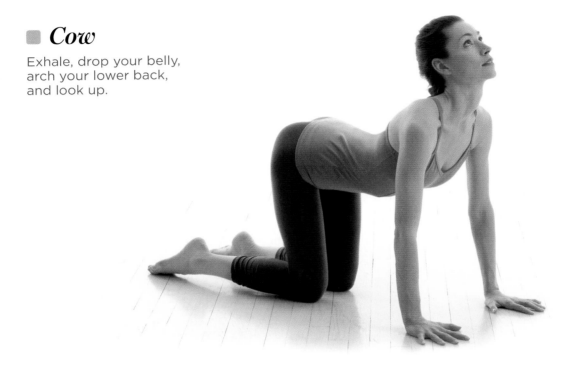

▪ *Sphinx*

Lie on your stomach. Bring your elbows
under your shoulders and rest your forearms on the floor in front of you. Spread
your fingers, press your hands against
the floor, and pull your upper arms gently
back toward your torso while keeping
your forearms where they are. Inhale and
press your chest forward, and bring your
shoulder blades together while dropping
them down and away from your ears.

*Drop your
shoulders
away from
your ears.*

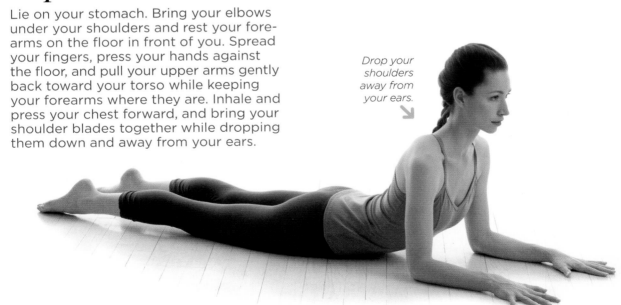

■ *Up Dog*

Keeping your palms pressed down, straighten your arms, roll your shoulders down and back, and press your chest forward. Let your thighs and shins come up off the floor.

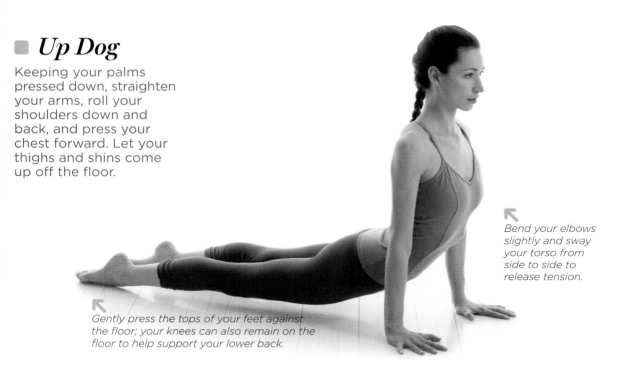

Bend your elbows slightly and sway your torso from side to side to release tension.

Gently press the tops of your feet against the floor; your knees can also remain on the floor to help support your lower back.

■ *Bow*

Lying on your belly, bend your knees and grab the outside of your feet. Gently press your feet into your hands and lift your chest and knees up. Keep the back of your neck long.

TIP: *If holding your ankles in bow pose hurts your back or knees, try this more gentle variation instead: Lie flat on your stomach with your arms down along your sides. Lift your chest forward and up while extending your legs straight back. Raise your feet off the floor straight behind you. Take 5 long, deep breaths and gently lower yourself.*

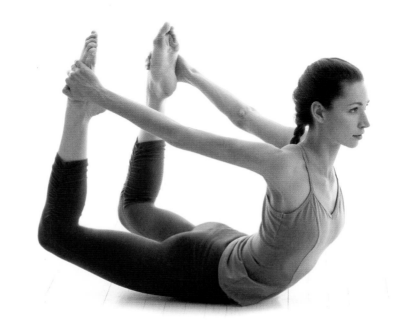

Main POSE

Tabletop

From a sitting position with your knees bent and feet flat on the floor, place your hands on the floor a few inches behind your hips, fingers facing toward you. Inhale, press up, and lift your torso until it's parallel to the floor.

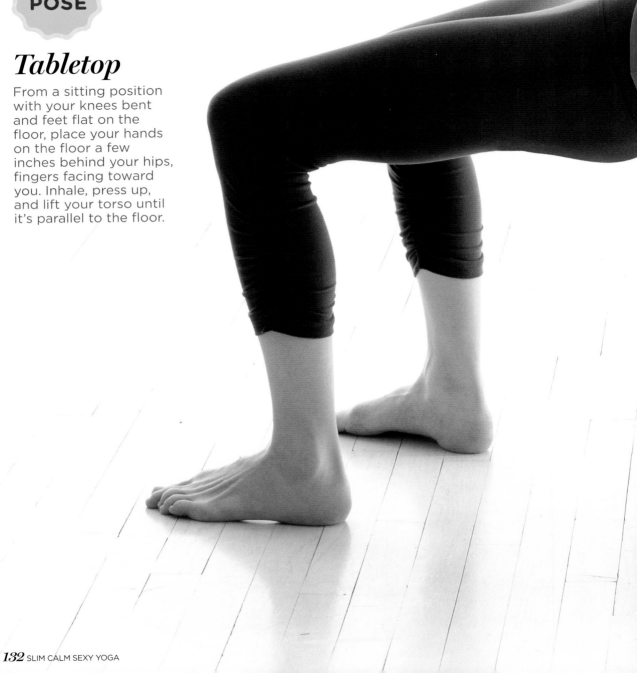

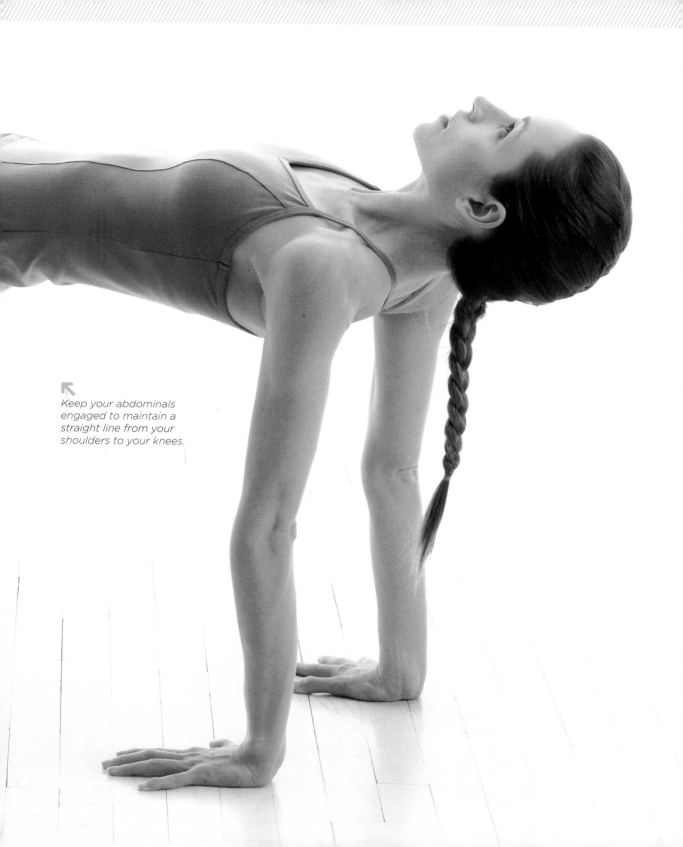

Keep your abdominals engaged to maintain a straight line from your shoulders to your knees.

Baby Bridge

Lie down on your back with your knees bent and feet flat on the floor. Place your hands on the floor next to your hips and gently lift your hips, pressing your arms into the floor. Grab your ankles with your hands.

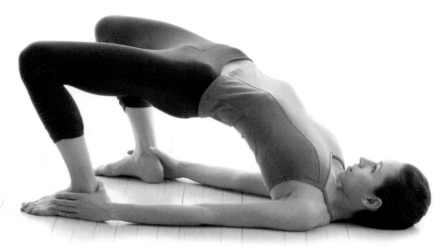

Bridge, Hands Interlaced

Lace your fingers together between your feet. Wiggle your shoulder blades together and press your chest toward your chin. Keep your feet flat on the floor and reach your hips up farther.

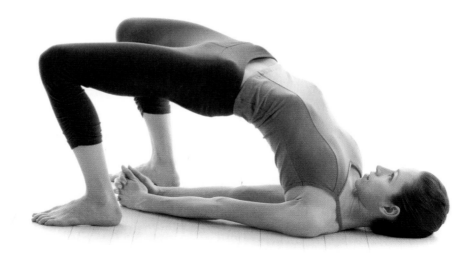

Supported Bridge on One Block

Place a block vertically on your mat. Lie down, bend your knees, and lift your hips so you're resting the small of your back on the block. Rest your head on the floor and relax your arms out to the sides.

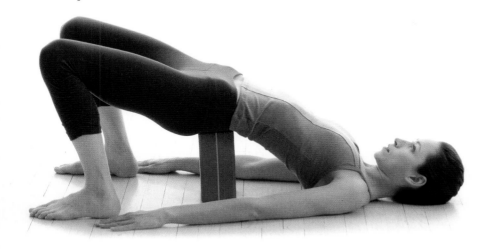

Supported Bridge on Two Blocks

Place a block lengthwise on its side on your mat. Lie down, resting the middle of your spine along the center of the block. Stand the other block vertically and place it under your lower back. Let your arms rest at your sides.

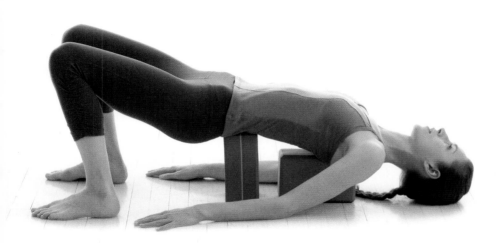

■ *Back-to-Back Sitting*

Sit back to back, either on the floor or on a block, in a comfortable cross-legged position. Rest your palms on your thighs and extend your spine upward. Lean back slightly against your partner. Close your eyes and follow your breath for a few minutes.

PARTNER-SUPPORTED POSES
Practicing yoga with

your partner is a great way to spend time together. Any time you support each other while performing a physical endeavor, you build trust and communication, which can help strengthen your relationship. When practicing these poses, make sure to switch roles each time so you both get the benefits.

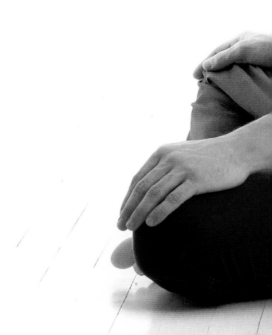

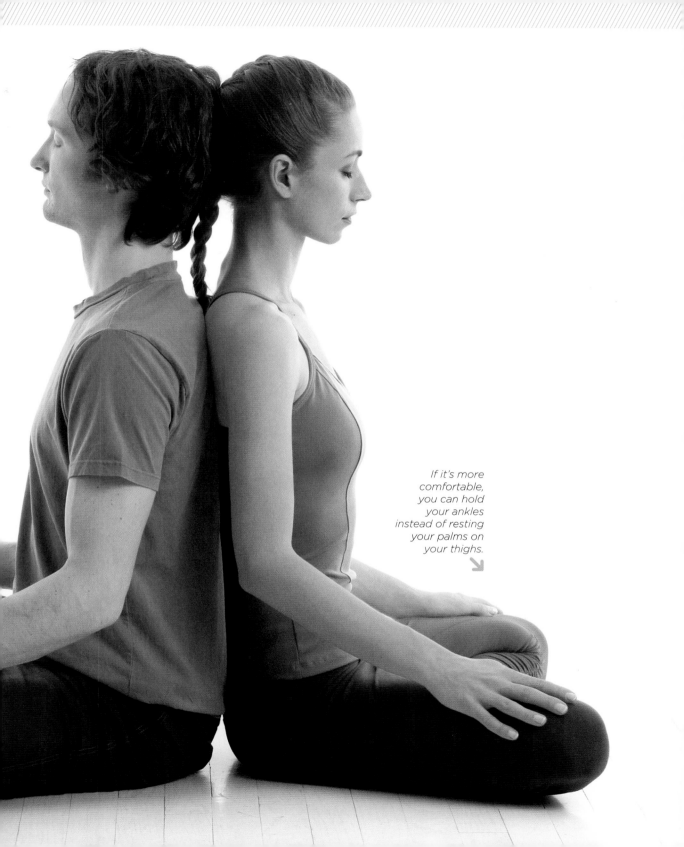

If it's more comfortable, you can hold your ankles instead of resting your palms on your thighs.

Back-to-Back Lean

Sit up tall with the soles of your feet together. Lean back against each other. Breathe here for a few breaths. Allow your hips to release each time you exhale.

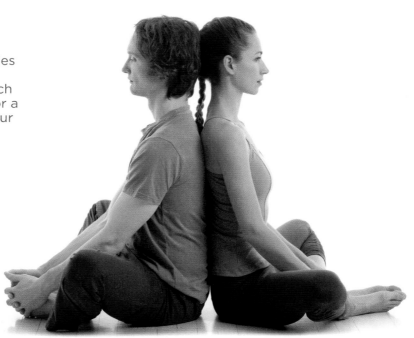

Back-to-Back Twist

Sit up tall. Place your left hand on your right knee and your right hand on your partner's left thigh, just above the knee. He should do the same. Press down on each other's thighs and twist your torsos to the right. On each inhale, lift up a little higher in your torso. On each exhale, twist a little farther.

You can hold onto your left foot with your left hand instead of resting it on your knee.

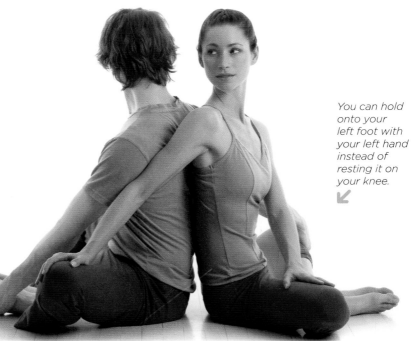

Back-to-Back Recline

From your back-to-back position, lean back on your partner, resting your head on his upper back, while he bends forward. Stay here for 5 long, deep breaths, then switch.

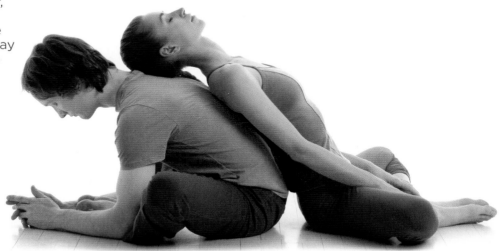

JUST GO WITH IT

Don't try to force a "perfect couple" moment. Stay with your breath and stay open, and whatever happens will be authentic.

■ *Seated Straddle*

Face each other and spread your legs wide. Depending on how flexible each of you is, you can place your feet together, or if one partner is less flexible, that partner can place his or her feet at the other's ankles or calves. Link hands, wrists, or arms and breathe here for a few breaths.

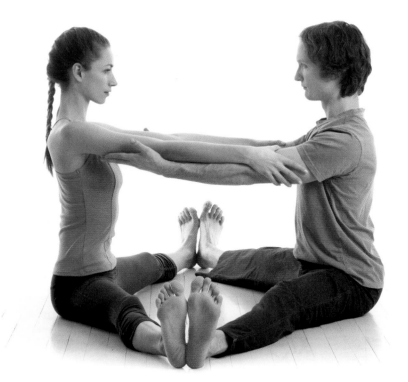

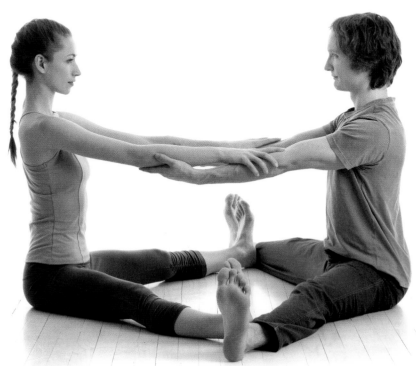

Forward Bend Back Press

Sit with your backs together, your legs stretched straight or slightly bent in front of you, and your feet flexed. Take turns coming into an easy forward bend. The partner not bending forward places his or her feet on the floor and sits gently on the other person's lower back. Ease into how much weight you're resting on your partner, and remember to communicate about how it feels.

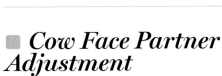

Cow Face Partner Adjustment

Have your partner sit on the mat in cow phase pose resting his forearms on the floor. Kneel on your left leg behind him and extend your right leg behind you, toes under. Press your chest against his upper back, gently guiding his torso forward.

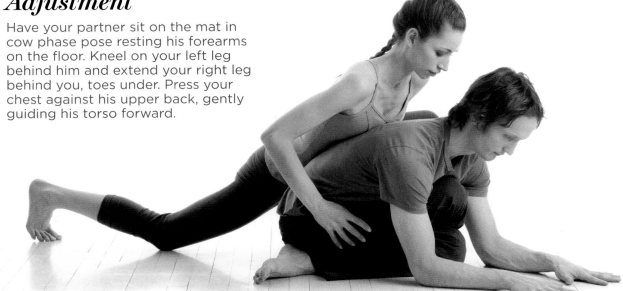

Eagle Twist Partner Adjustment

Have your partner lie on his back, hooking his right foot around the outside of his left calf. He should bend his knees and let them fall to the left. Stand on the mat below his hips and place your right hand just above the outside of his right knee and your left hand on his right shoulder. He should exhale while you press down and inhale when you ease the pressure.

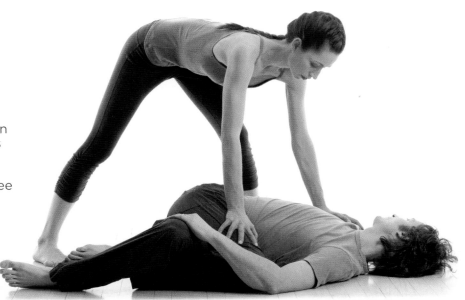

Corpse Partner Adjustment

Have your partner lie on his back in corpse pose, eyes closed. Stand over his legs and place your right hand under his left lower back and your left hand on top of his right thigh. Gently lift his lower back while pressing down on his thigh.

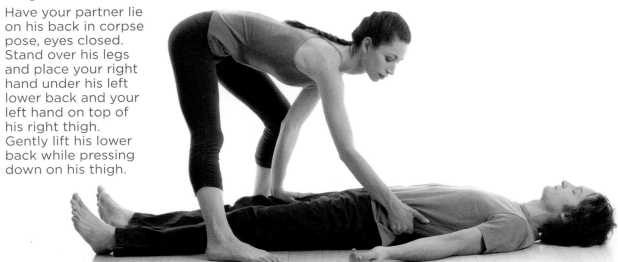

Corpse Neck Massage

While your partner is in corpse pose, kneel down behind his head, place your hands at the base of his neck, and alternate moving each hand toward his head, rubbing his neck as you go.

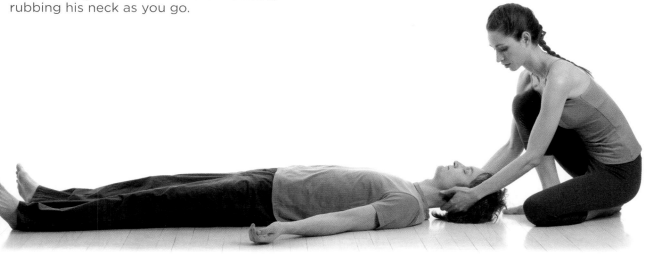

Corpse Temple Massage

While your partner is in corpse pose, kneel down behind his head, place your fingertips on the center of his forehead, right above his eyebrows, and gently press down and out toward his temples. When you reach his temples, press a little more firmly.

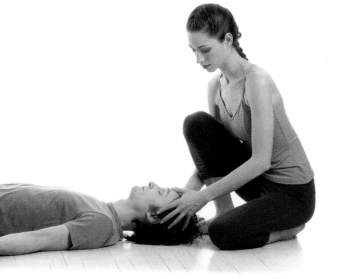

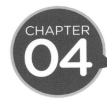

CHAPTER
04

slim
yoga

The secret to taking
control of your weight

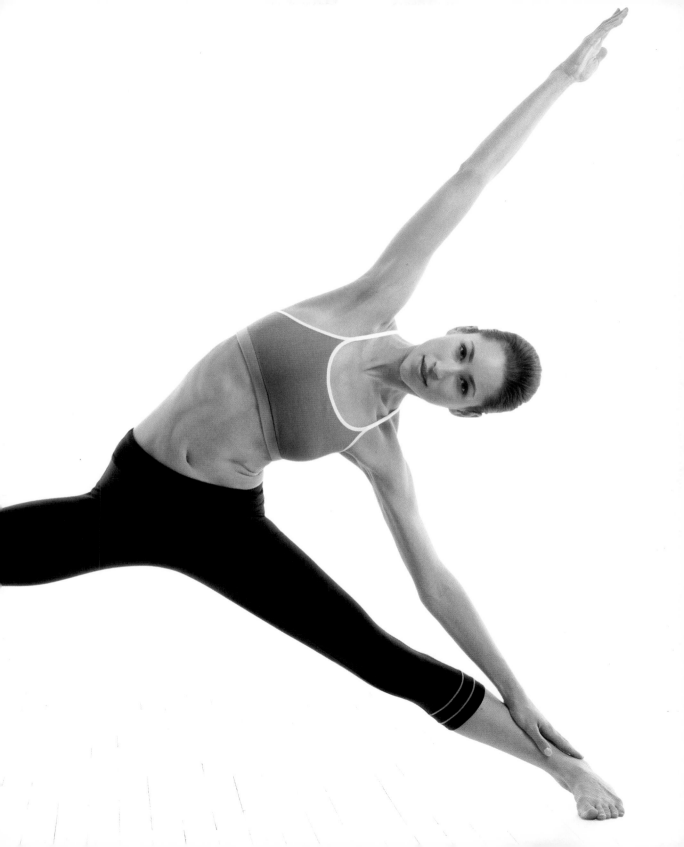

Everyone

knows that diets and workout plans are useless unless you stick to them. To get slim-body results, you have to first understand that losing weight and maintaining a healthy physique require a complete lifestyle makeover.

Sounds daunting, huh?

It doesn't have to be.

This is where the principles of yoga come in. Doing yoga will give you great muscle tone and flexibility, for sure. But by managing your stress and putting you in touch with your body's needs, yoga can play a starring role in your slim-body lifestyle overhaul.

I'm guessing this won't come as a shock to you, but I'm going to put it out there anyway: Stress is directly linked to packing on pounds.

In an American Psychological Association survey of more than 1,800 people, 43 percent of respondents admitted to overeating or to eating unhealthy foods in response to stress. And women were more likely to do it than men were.

Take a minute to wrap your head around the concept of "your body on stress." Stress is like your own personal bodyguard that launches into defense mode in the face of a threat. At the center of this effort are your adrenal glands, which protect you by unleashing the hormones cortisol and adrenaline.

As the fight-or-flight hormone, adrenaline gives you an instant megashot of energy so you can face down a conflict or get away from it altogether. But cortisol is more like an overprotective mother whose sole mission is to feed and nurture you. And it's the reason you want to stuff your face during a freak-out.

Cortisol's effects are hard to miss: It makes you want to eat everything in sight, and the easier to digest, the better. That's because it requires foods high in fat and sugar, energy sources your body can access fast. Some scientists believe that cortisol also messes with the signals that control appetite and feelings of fullness, which is why being stressed out may make you crave dessert even after a big dinner. Storing up reserve energy (in the form of excess poundage) was supremely helpful back when stress was about life or death, and when we burned through thousands of calories collecting food, building fires, or fleeing scary beasts. Not so much anymore, now that stress is more about sitting at a computer plowing through a mammoth to-do list.

To make matters worse, when stress causes your cortisol levels to stay chronically high, it can have long-term detrimental effects on your weight. That's because the hormone encourages your body to store fat—in your belly especially—rather than burn it. It's how nature makes sure you don't starve when food is scarce and that you have backup energy stores for handling life-threatening situations.

Problem is, abdominal fat has both a greater blood supply (an express lane for cortisol) and more receptors for the hormone. Cortisol also reduces the production of testosterone, which is essential for muscle building. Chronically low testosterone can cause you to lose muscle mass, which ultimately slows your metabolism.

Exercise, including yoga, is proven

to reduce cortisol levels and weight. In 2005, researchers measured cortisol levels in female volunteers who then participated in 3 months of yoga classes. Afterward, the women had significantly lower cortisol levels compared with women who didn't do yoga. And a study published in the journal *Alternative Therapies in Health and Medicine* found that people who practiced yoga regularly for 4 years or more actually gained less weight over time than those who did no yoga. What's more, the overweight subjects in the study managed to lose weight over a 10-year period.

You'd be pretty well set in the slim department if yoga's weight-loss influence stopped there. But the fat-fighting power of yoga goes even further. Perhaps the most lasting and far-reaching benefit of yoga is the awareness, or mindfulness, it teaches you. Once you make yoga a regular part of your life, you'll notice a newfound awareness of your body and mind. And from that awareness blossoms an intuitive sense of your abilities and limits, along with what's good for you and what's not. For instance, you begin to know when to push harder in a pose and when to back off, as well as which foods to eat and which ones to avoid.

In studies on what causes obesity, researchers have found that overweight people often are clueless about their eating and exercise habits; they tend to underestimate how much they eat while overestimating their activity. (Sometimes I think it's just easier to blame something you can't control than to recognize what you can and take action to address it. How many times have you heard a friend say, "I have a slow metabolism" or "I have fat genes"? Maybe you've even said it yourself.)

The *New England Journal of Medicine* once published a fascinating study on this phenomenon. Researchers tracked the diet and exercise habits of people who claimed they couldn't lose weight even though they cut calories. The upshot was that the volunteers had dramatically underreported their calories by 47 percent and overreported their activity by 51 percent. And when researchers compared their ability to burn calories with that of a control group, there was zero difference. Their failed "diets" had nothing to do with sluggish metabolisms; they didn't work because the people had no idea they were eating too much and not moving enough!

Awareness is a powerful thing. And once you hone it, you're better able to discern what your body and mind need to be healthy. For example, maybe you'll start to notice how great your food tastes, and then you'll slow down so you can savor every delicious bite—which is a good thing, because research has found that when you take your time at the table, you eat less. Scientists at the University of Rhode Island had 30 volunteers eat two identical meals in a lab. During one, they were told basically to shovel the food down with a soupspoon. At the other, they were instructed to eat with a tea-spoon, pause between bites, and chew each mouthful 20 to 30 times. The volunteers practically inhaled the first meal in a zippy 9 minutes, on average. But when they lingered over their food, the meal stretched to nearly 30 minutes—and here's the kicker: They ate 10 percent less. Researchers believe that when you eat more slowly, your body has more time to register fullness, so you stop feeling hungry before you dive into a second—or third!—helping.

Along with lowering your stress levels and toning your muscles, practicing yoga will cultivate a power of awareness you may not have known you had; one that holds the key to getting the slim, sexy body you want. The following routines build mindful-ness and help rein in cortisol so you can eat healthfully, kick-start your metabolism, and burn fat effectively.

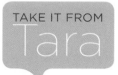

TAKE IT FROM
Tara

GOALS
VERSUS
INTENTIONS

It's worth recognizing the difference between setting goals and setting intentions. In the yogic tradition, intention is something you can control. An intention related to weight loss could be, "I will have only one glass of wine with dinner," or "I'll eat just a bite of dessert"—which is more realistic than "I will lose 10 pounds." After all, you have control over what you do, not what your weight does.

A.M. Metabolism Kickoff

Starting the day with 5 minutes of yoga will calm your nervous system, focus your mind, and rev up your metabolism. Do this on your mat or from the comfort of your bed, and take advantage of the fresh moment you wake up, before your mind starts racing with all you have planned for the day. Practice this three times a week for the best results.

the ROUTINE *Try the following sequence, staying in each pose for 5 deep inhales and exhales, unless otherwise noted.*

■ **Lying-Down V**
p. 117

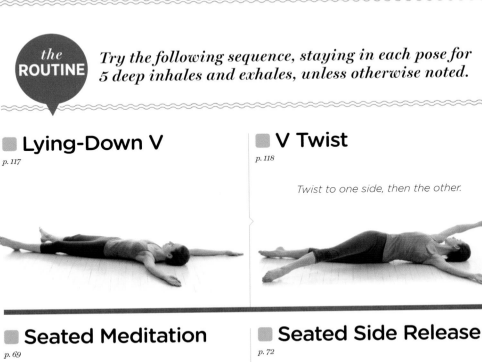

■ **V Twist**
p. 118

Twist to one side, then the other.

■ **Seated Meditation**
p. 69

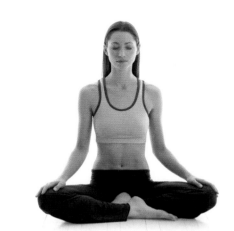

■ **Seated Side Release**
p. 72

Reach to one side, then the other.

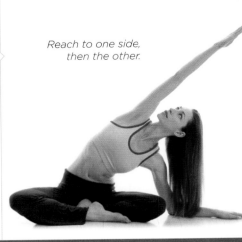

Knee-to-Chest Circle

p. 118

Start with the one knee, then do the other. Softly roll onto one side and take a few deep breaths. Let your whole body relax, and use your exhales to send away any tension that tries to creep in.

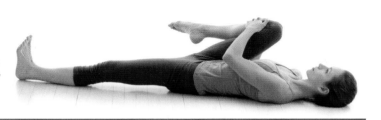

Seated Palm Press

p. 71

Standing Palm Press

p. 29

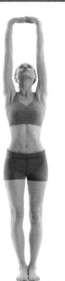

Exhale and carefully lower your arms down by your sides.

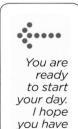

You are ready to start your day. I hope you have a great one!

Fat Burning

A sure way to fry fat on the mat is to move your body through challenging poses that call upon all your muscles to work in novel ways. Practice this routine four times a week for best results. Keep a towel by your side; you will sweat!

the ROUTINE

Try the following sequence, staying in each pose for 5 deep inhales and exhales, unless otherwise noted.

▪ Plank
p. 95

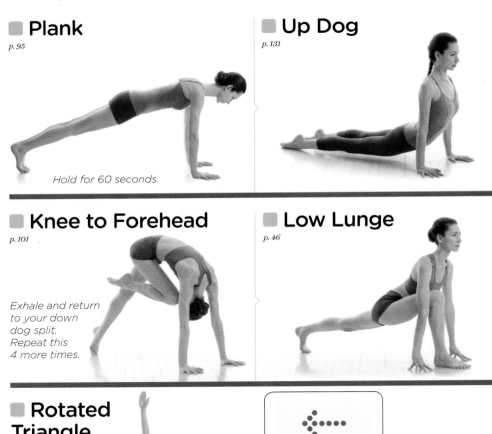

Hold for 60 seconds.

▪ Up Dog
p. 131

▪ Knee to Forehead
p. 101

Exhale and return to your down dog split. Repeat this 4 more times.

▪ Low Lunge
p. 46

▪ Rotated Triangle
p. 57

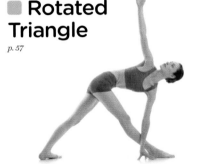

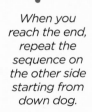

When you reach the end, repeat the sequence on the other side starting from down dog.

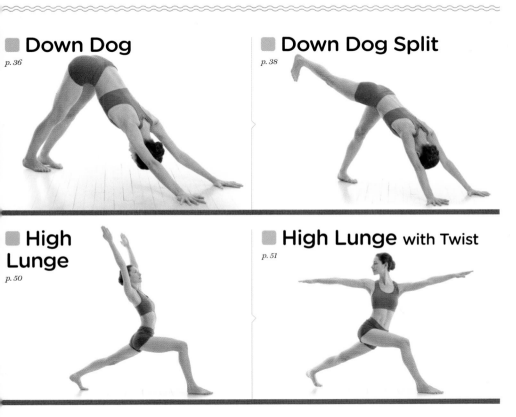

■ Down Dog
p. 36

■ Down Dog Split
p. 38

■ High Lunge
p. 50

■ High Lunge **with Twist**
p. 51

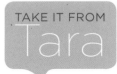

TAKE IT FROM
Tara

THE
POWER
OF PLANK

Holding plank pose for a full minute can be a serious challenge. Long, deep breaths help the seconds tick by faster, so try to guide your breath back to long and deep if you start to panic and it becomes short and fast. If you need a break, try pressing up to down dog for a breath or two and then coming back into your plank instead of giving up or collapsing your hips toward the floor. Staying in the pose, especially when your mind would prefer something easier, builds the strength and focus you need to reach any goal.

Metabolism Revving

The poses in this routine draw on your strength, and holding them will get your heart rate up to rev your metabolism. The ancient yogis believed that practicing shoulder stand stimulates your thyroid and parathyroid glands in the neck by combining inversion with constriction between the chin and neck, followed by release. They also believed that this movement brings more blood flow to the region, improves overall circulation, and regulates metabolism. Even if you think you have a sluggish metabolism, practicing this routine twice a week will keep it humming—and help you burn calories all day.

the **ROUTINE**

Try the following sequence, staying in each pose for 5 deep inhales and exhales.

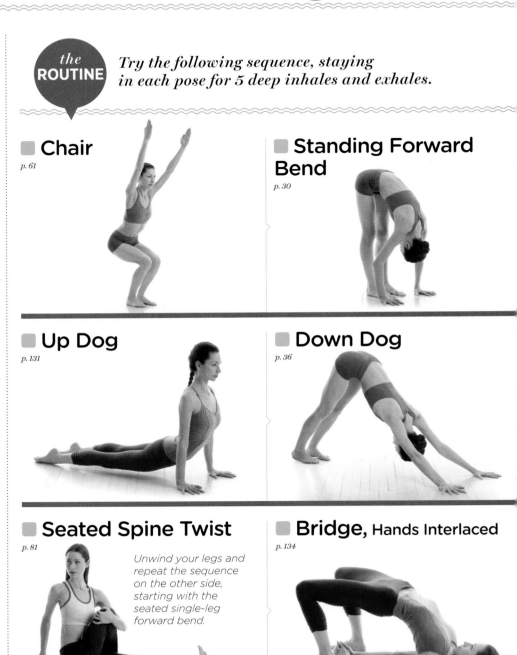

■ **Chair**
p. 61

■ **Standing Forward Bend**
p. 30

■ **Up Dog**
p. 131

■ **Down Dog**
p. 36

■ **Seated Spine Twist**
p. 81

Unwind your legs and repeat the sequence on the other side, starting with the seated single-leg forward bend.

■ **Bridge,** Hands Interlaced
p. 134

▪ Plank
p. 95

▪ Half Pushup
p. 96

▸▸▸▸▸▸

Jump your legs forward and repeat the above sequence 4 times, then move on to the next sequence.

▪ Seated Single-Leg Forward Bend
p. 79

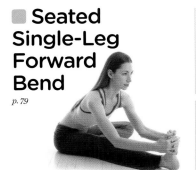

▪ Seated Shin Hug
p. 80

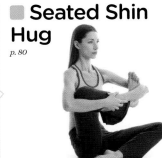

▪ Plow
p. 112

▪ Shoulder Stand
p. 114

Try shoulder stand only if you are comfortable in plow.

TAKE IT FROM

Tara

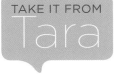

PINBALL WIZARD

Spending a little extra time in up dog can release tension in all areas of your back. Keep rolling your shoulders together behind you and dropping them down and away from your ears. Try swaying your torso from side to side between your arms, and breathe deeply into any tight areas. You can do this each time you come into an up dog, if it feels good to your spine. At the studio we call this one "pinballing your torso between your arms" (because it looks like a pinball machine when the whole class is doing it together).

Toning / Full Body

Maybe you've recently slimmed down and want to add definition to your muscles now that they're not hidden under a layer of fat. Or maybe you've always been thin but want more tone. Sleek, sculpted muscle is a direct result of consistent practice. To get results, it's important to challenge your body to move beyond your comfort zone. The next sequence works your entire body, and the ones that follow focus on individual parts—abs, lower body, and upper body—leaving you with a healthy, sexy physique. Depending on your goals, practice each routine four times a week.

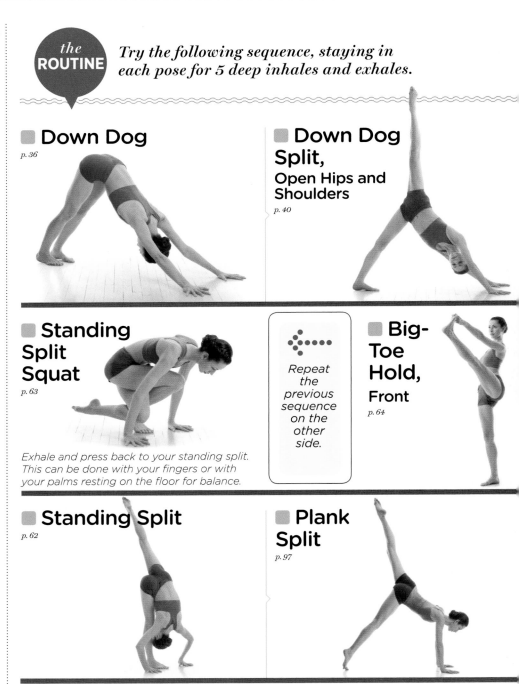

the ROUTINE *Try the following sequence, staying in each pose for 5 deep inhales and exhales.*

■ Down Dog
p. 36

■ Down Dog Split,
Open Hips and Shoulders
p. 40

■ Standing Split Squat
p. 63

Exhale and press back to your standing split. This can be done with your fingers or with your palms resting on the floor for balance.

Repeat the previous sequence on the other side.

■ Big-Toe Hold,
Front
p. 64

■ Standing Split
p. 62

■ Plank Split
p. 97

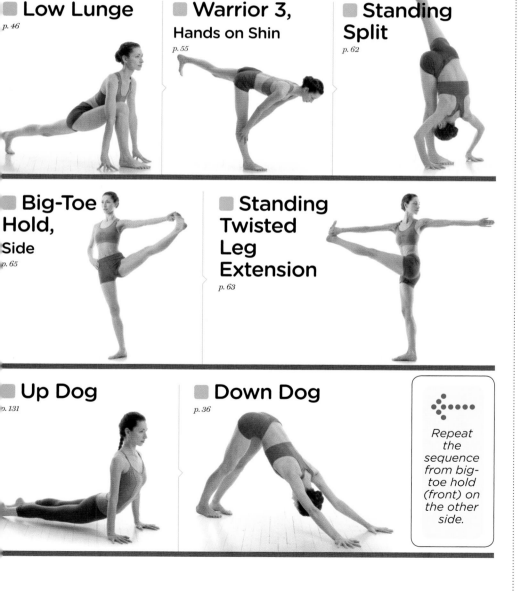

■ Low Lunge
p. 46

■ Warrior 3,
Hands on Shin
p. 55

■ Standing Split
p. 62

■ Big-Toe Hold,
Side
p. 65

■ Standing Twisted Leg Extension
p. 63

■ Up Dog
p. 131

■ Down Dog
p. 36

Repeat the sequence from big-toe hold (front) on the other side.

TAKE IT FROM
Tara

STAY ON THE BUS!

We have a saying at Strala: "Stay on the bus." If you are in the middle of a sequence that you find ridiculously challenging, stay with it. Even if you're not doing the full extension of the pose, it's more beneficial to stick with it in some way than to quit and wait until the next pose. If you fall out of a pose, take your time and move back into it with care and attention. When you stay on the bus, you challenge yourself to get stronger physically and mentally.

Toning /Abs

Sure, a toned tummy is great for showing off at the beach, but having a strong core also makes fat burning, strength building and balance more efficient. Take your whole practice to the next level by making a few core moves a priority.

the **ROUTINE**

Try the following sequence, staying in each pose for 5 deep inhales and exhales, unless otherwise noted.

■ Leg Raise with Block
p. 123

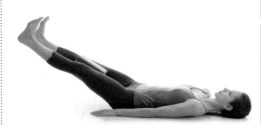

■ Feet Up with Block
p. 122

Return to the previous pose, then repeat up-and-down movement 20 times.

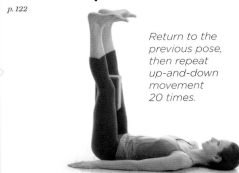

■ Hamstring Release
p. 119

Do to one side, then the other.

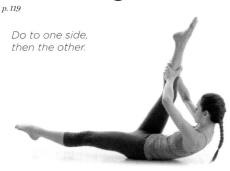

■ Knee Cross
p. 120

Do to one side, then the other.

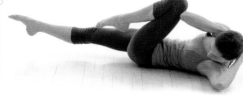

Bent Boat

p. 82

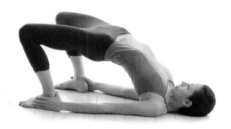

Hover with Block

p. 124

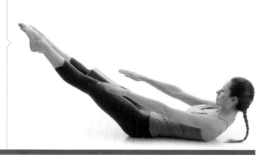

Baby Bridge

p. 134

Toning / Lower Body

Prepare to drop the words "problem areas" from your vocabulary. These poses will lift, shape, and carve your body into the form you're after. Shaping up a sexy lower half doesn't have to be a tireless battle. Bring on the short shorts! Calorie burning and toning are two big elements that factor into developing a sexy bum and thighs. Moving with your breath through challenging yoga poses will get the calories sweating off. Targeting the big muscle groups will cultivate lots of strength and tone. This routine will shed excess inches and shape up the rest.

the ROUTINE *Try the following sequence, staying in each pose for 5 deep inhales and exhales, unless otherwise noted.*

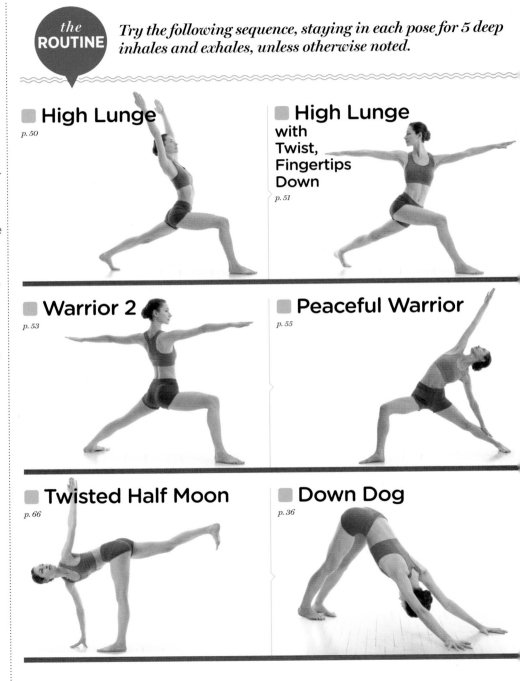

■ **High Lunge**
p. 50

■ **High Lunge with Twist, Fingertips Down**
p. 51

■ **Warrior 2**
p. 53

■ **Peaceful Warrior**
p. 55

■ **Twisted Half Moon**
p. 66

■ **Down Dog**
p. 36

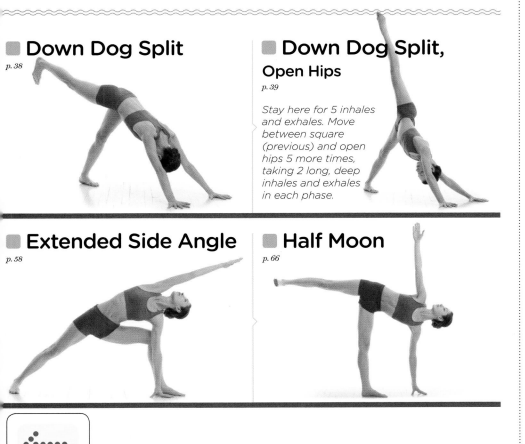

■ Down Dog Split
p. 38

■ Down Dog Split,
Open Hips
p. 39

Stay here for 5 inhales and exhales. Move between square (previous) and open hips 5 more times, taking 2 long, deep inhales and exhales in each phase.

■ Extended Side Angle
p. 58

■ Half Moon
p. 66

Repeat the entire sequence on the other side.

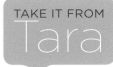

KEEP IT FRESH

Stay active in your poses. You want to keep a small amount of movement when you are holding a pose to get the most benefits. This is different from fidgeting or nervous adjustment. Instead, use your breathing to lengthen tight areas, lift some of the effort out of difficult positions, and sink a little deeper into open spaces. If you had to stay in the pose for 30 minutes, how would you keep it fresh?

Toning / Upper Body

This series will work your arms, shoulders, upper back, and chest—hard. Feel free to take a moment or two to shake out your arms between poses.

the ROUTINE

Try the following sequence, staying in each pose for 5 deep inhales and exhales, unless otherwise noted.

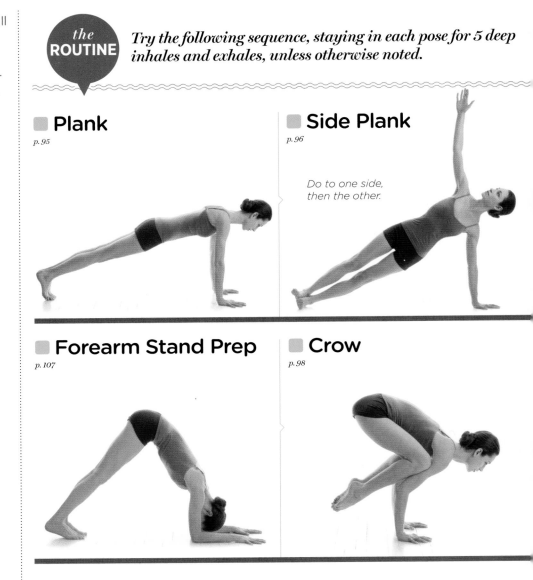

Plank
p. 95

Side Plank
p. 96

Do to one side, then the other.

Forearm Stand Prep
p. 107

Crow
p. 98

Down Dog
p. 36

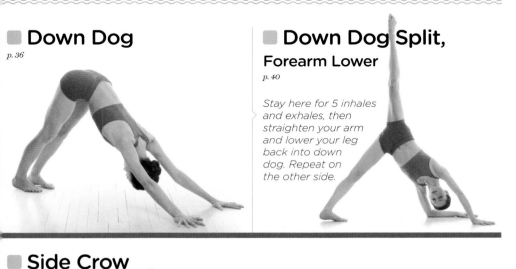

Down Dog Split,
Forearm Lower
p. 40

Stay here for 5 inhales and exhales, then straighten your arm and lower your leg back into down dog. Repeat on the other side.

Side Crow
p. 100

Do to one side, then the other.

BREATHE DEEP

Check in on your breath. During challenging sequences, it's easy to lose track of long, deep breathing. If your breaths become short and fast, guide them back to long and deep. Deep breathing will help you through a challenging routine like this one. When you breathe short and fast, your body switches into panic mode and tightens up. When you take long, deep breaths, your body and mind remain calm, and you're able to move with control. By getting rid of unnecessary anxiety and tension, deep breathing can help you move well past whatever limitations you might think you have.

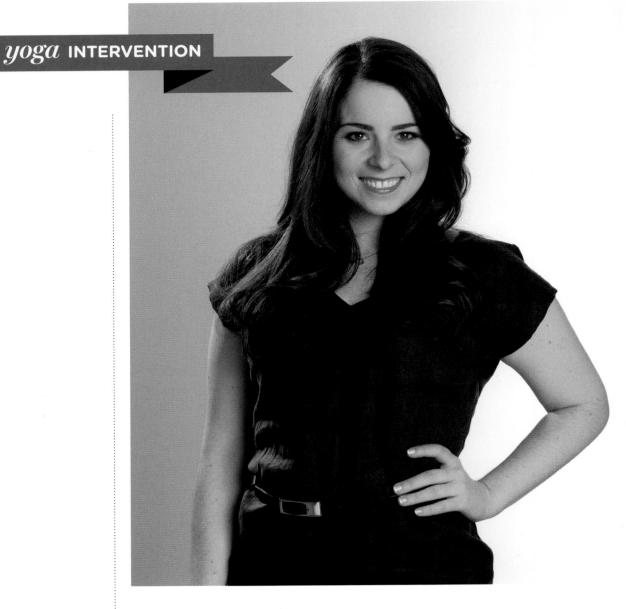

Fernanda Hess

THE ISSUE: STRESS EATING AND WEIGHT GAIN

"Breathing consciously during yoga movements connects my mind to my body and keeps me focused on the present. It resets the thinking patterns that get me in trouble with food—fear, anxiety, sadness—which usually relate to my past or future, never my present. So if I keep myself in the present, I am happy. I make better decisions about food and my life."

Brazilian native Fernanda Hess has always had to watch her diet to maintain a normal weight. "It's been a constant struggle over the years," admits the 26-year-old, "especially during times of stress."

The problem came to a head when Fernanda moved from Rio de Janeiro to Boston in 2004 to attend college. The combination of relocating, experiencing college life, and adapting to a new culture was beyond stressful. "I used food to cope," Fernanda says, and her weight skyrocketed from 120 to 155 pounds during her first semester. On her 5-foot-5-inch frame, the extra heft was hard to ignore. "The change in my body really upset me," she admits.

"I began walking, running, and lifting weights," Fernanda says. "I even worked with a personal trainer." But it was a lot of effort with little result. "Even though I was burning 500 to 600 extra calories a day, I could not control my impulse to eat," she says. "Maybe I lost 7 pounds."

The gym also offered yoga classes, and one day when Fernanda's stress was out of control, she tried one to see if it would help her relax. "The class was extremely challeng-ing, but afterward I felt amazing and came back the next day for another one," she says.

After a few sessions, Fernanda realized her compulsion to eat was starting to diminish, and eventually she ditched train-ing altogether for yoga. "In 8 months, I lost 35 pounds," she says.

"Yoga makes me feel con-nected to my body in a way that helps me control what I eat," a fact that would be confirmed just a few years later in 2009, when Fernanda moved to New York City to start a new job as a voice and speech coach and she stopped going to class. The re-sult? She regained 17 pounds. "I guess I don't react well to mov-ing!" she says. Once Fernanda settled into her job, determined not to go through a repeat of her "freshman 35," she got back on her yoga mat and made regu-lar practice a priority. Within a month, she'd lost 5 pounds. "Yoga does amazing things for my impulse control when it comes to eating," she says.

calm yoga

Om improvements for maximum chill

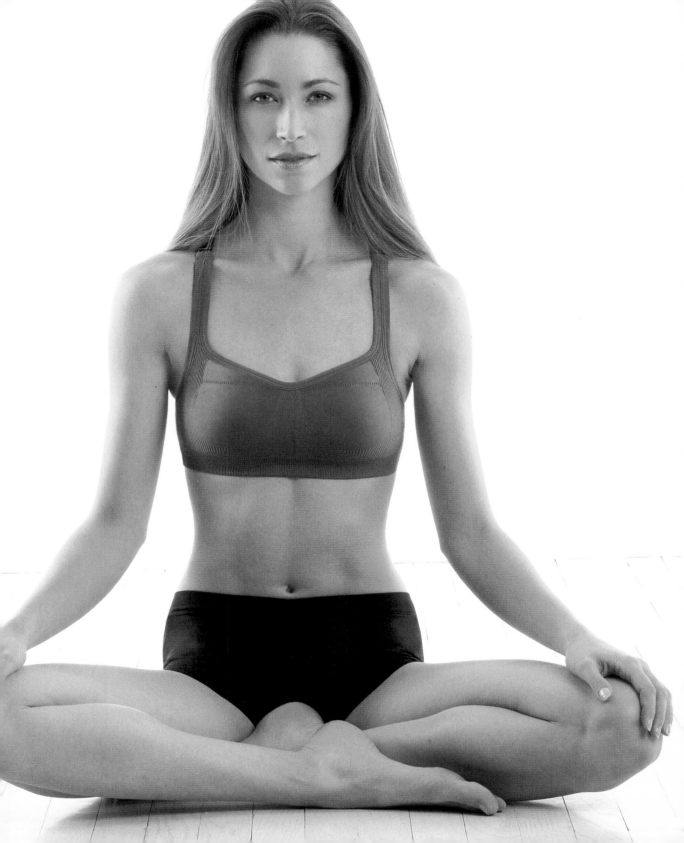

In the previous chapter,

I talked a lot about the connection between stress and weight. But stress messes with a lot more than your middle. It has a negative effect on so many other parts of your life, including your health, which makes it that much more important to control.

Stress is like the laundry. It will always be there, and if you don't deal with it regularly, it gets out of control. Skip the laundry and the resulting mountain of dirty clothes makes it impossible to find anything to wear. Avoid dealing with stress and you develop a frazzled mind prone to outbursts and meltdowns, making it impossible to deal with any challenge, from little bumps in the road to major life decisions.

Of all the things yoga can do for you, chilling you out is probably the benefit that's easiest to grasp. After all, even if you've done yoga only once in your life, I'm sure you felt the bliss as you lay prone in corpse pose at the end of class. So it's no surprise that yoga's effect on mental health is one of its most studied benefits. A few examples:

In 2009, researchers at Harvard Medical School looked at the effects of yoga and meditation on performance anxiety in a group of young professional musicians. (As a former dancer, I know from experience how anxiety can psychologically cripple a performer, regardless of skill or experience!) Subjects who took part in a 2-month program of yoga and meditation reported significantly fewer episodes of performance anxiety, general anxiety and tension, depression, and anger.

Researchers believe that by reducing stress and anxiety, practicing yoga actually affects the way your body responds to stress—lowering your heart rate and blood pressure and regulating your breathing. It may also increase heart rate variability, which helps your body better react to stressful situations.

In 2008, researchers at the University of Utah presented results from a study on yoga and pain. (People who have a low tolerance for pain are also more prone to stress.) The scientists used MRIs to watch how participants' brains physically reacted to pain and stress. The results were exciting because they showed an unequivocal physical result of yoga on the body's stress-management system: Not only did the subjects who practiced yoga exhibit the highest tolerance for pain, but their MRIs also showed the lowest pain-related brain activity.

In 2005, German researchers asked 24 women who described themselves as emotionally distressed to take two 90-minute yoga classes a week for 3 months. Women in a control group were told not to begin an exercise or stress-reduction program during the study period. At the end of the study, the women in the yoga group reported less stress, depression, anxiety, and fatigue, along with improved energy and well-being.

I could list study after study showing how yoga will improve your mental state, but it would fill an entire book. Besides, I suspect you know intuitively that even the simple act of resting your attention on your breath, instead of following your racing thoughts, has the power to bring you back to your center. Whether you are mildly stressed from daily tasks or dealing with tons of anxiety, the techniques in this chapter can take the edge off and get you back to feeling calm and focused. Improved sleep, less anxiety, and a boost in energy are just some of the benefits you'll enjoy.

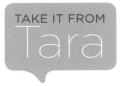

TAKE IT FROM
Tara

MAKE TIME

Tell me you haven't found yourself thinking that you'll slow down and destress when you find the time. How crazy is that? If you haven't "found" the time yet, you're not going to. You have to make the time. Start with 30 seconds here and there, then gradually make longer practice a priority.

Anxiety

We've all had symptoms of anxiety at some point in our lives: Sunday-night insomnia, butterflies before a first date, a racing heart during a meeting with the boss. Whether you're raising a family, working toward advancement in your career, or pursuing a degree, anxiety can find a way to ruin a big moment or make a goal that much harder to reach. Not only that, but busy lives can make anxiety feel like a chronic condition. The fact is, you'll get things done more efficiently and feel less anxious if you take a few moments to unwind. Do this routine twice a week to release tension so you can find your way back to calm.

the **ROUTINE**

Try the following sequence, staying in each pose for 5 deep inhales and exhales, unless otherwise noted.

■ Standing Forward Bend, Neck Release
p. 31

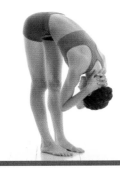

■ Squat Hang
p. 35

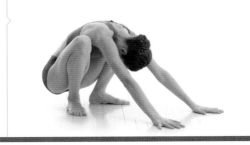

■ Boat Twist
p. 82

Stay here for 1 full inhale and exhale. Switch sides and repeat. Continue switching for 20 breaths.

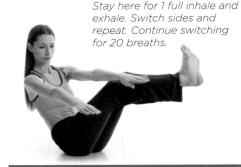

■ Tabletop
p. 132

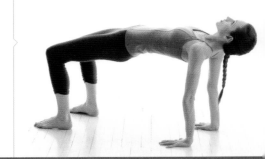

THE INDIAN MYSTIC KNOWN as Osho teaches that an anxious person feels separate from the world, with everyone conspiring against them. Trees and birds don't spend their days worrying; worry isn't helpful to them. It's also not helpful to us. Anxiety goes away with understanding. When we understand that existence takes care of all of us, we know that we are not only part of existence, we are essential to it. We see that the world is abundant. This is when life becomes a celebration and feelings of anxiety are recognized as foolish.

Crow

p. 98

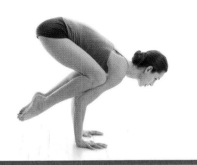

Squat Twist Bind

p. 35

Do to one side, then repeat on the other.

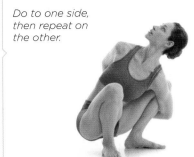

Seated Open-Leg Forward Bend

p. 78

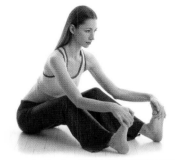

TAKE IT FROM
Tara

TAKE IT EASY

It's worth remembering that a little relaxing goes a long way. In yoga, it's optimal to use only the amount of energy you need to accomplish a pose. If you've been to yoga classes, I'm sure you've seen people working too hard to stay in a pose. Don't let that be you! If you maintain a strong work ethic, focus on the mat, and add relaxation to the mix, you'll be able to do more with less effort. (This practice goes a long way off the mat too, by the way.)

Depression

Many lab hours have been devoted to proving the strong connection between yoga and mood improvement for people who face situations that would make even the calmest among us crumble: women with breast cancer, people with epilepsy, and caregivers of dementia patients. A study published in the *Psychiatric Rehabilitation Journal* surveyed psychiatric patients on a variety of mental health symptoms, including depression, before and after they took a single yoga class. Their self-reported depression levels decreased after the class.

Everyone feels blue from time to time. Your situation may not be »

the ROUTINE *Try the following sequence, staying in each pose for 5 deep inhales and exhales, unless otherwise noted.*

Seated Meditation
p. 69

Stay here for 5 minutes.

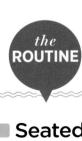

Seated Easy Twist
p. 73

Do to one side, then the other.

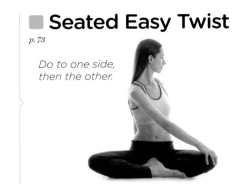

Standing Arm Reach
p. 28

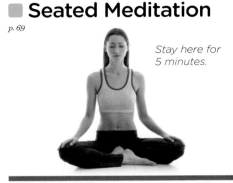

Standing Arch
p. 29

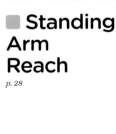

Standing Forward Bend, Calf Hold
p. 32

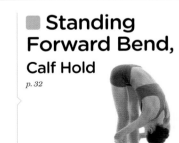

Warrior 1, Interlaced Hands, Shoulder Release
p. 53

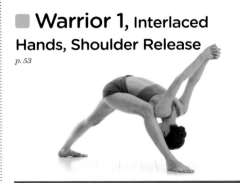

Down Dog
p. 36

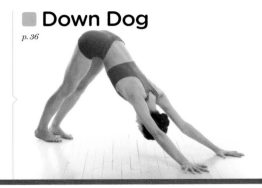

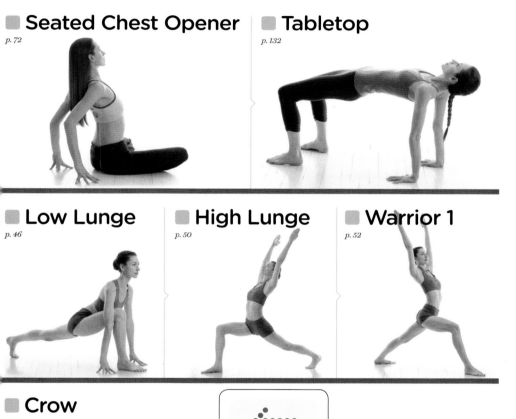

Seated Chest Opener
p. 72

Tabletop
p. 132

Low Lunge
p. 46

High Lunge
p. 50

Warrior 1
p. 52

Crow
p. 98

Go back to the low lunge, and with your left leg forward repeat the sequence on the other side.

>> as extreme as those of the subjects in most studies of yoga and depression, but if your feelings begin to dominate your life, things can seem out of control. Yoga and meditation can release stress from both your body and your mind, and according to research, can also raise endorphin levels, leaving you feeling lighter, happier, calmer, and more cen-tered. Moving may be the last thing you feel like doing when you're down, but knowing that a few simple practices can bring you back to your center may be a good incentive. Practice this routine twice a week to banish the blues.

Insomnia

Have you ever had problems sleeping? Are you exhausted but unable to get to sleep? Does your mind race at night? Do you get a rush of unwanted energy when you really want to fall asleep? If this sounds like you, I know how you feel, and you are not alone: The National Sleep Foundation estimates that three-quarters of Americans have problems sleeping several nights a week. The good news is, yoga can help. A 2009 study in the *International Medical Journal of Experimental and Clinical Research* found that after patients with sleep problems did two sessions of yoga and meditation during the day, the quality of »

the ROUTINE *Try the following sequence in bed, staying in each pose for 5 deep inhales and exhales, unless otherwise noted.*

Seated Meditation
p. 69

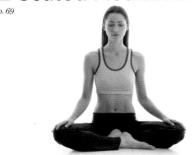

Sit up comfortably, with your legs either folded or straight in front of you—whichever is easier for you. Lean slightly back on your pillows or headboard. Close your eyes, rest your hands on your thighs, and just breathe here for a few minutes. This doesn't have to be a serious meditation—it's just a short while to do nothing but breathe.

Seated Forward Bend
p. 74

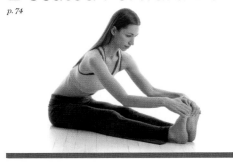

Seated Forward Bend, Round Back
p. 76

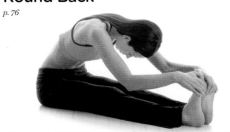

Half Happy Baby
p. 119

Do one leg, then the other.

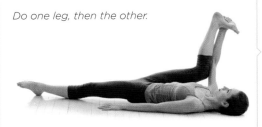

Spine Twist
p. 125

Twist to one side, then the other.

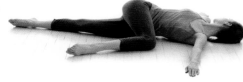

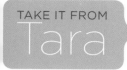

TAKE IT FROM
Tara

SLEEP SECRETS

Shut off the computer and TV when it gets close to bedtime. The bright screen can overstimulate your mind and add to restlessness. Try to create a routine for yourself before bed, finishing with this yoga sequence and then a good night's sleep. Whether it's getting into your favorite pj's and brushing your teeth or just giving yourself a certain block of time with your favorite book, routines help your body and brain prepare for what you want them to do.

Seated Easy Twist

p. 73

Do to one side, then the other.

Seated Cross-Legged Easy Forward Bend

p. 79

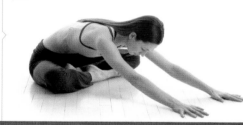

Knee to Chest

p. 124

Do one leg, then the other.

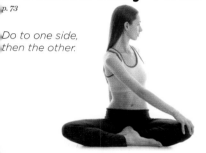

Single Leg Extension

p. 125

Extend one leg, then the other. This will help you drop any tension left in your body before bed.

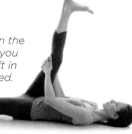

V Twist

p. 118

Twist to one side, then the other.

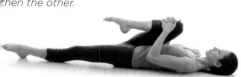

Corpse

p. 126

Take a few deep breaths into your abdomen and exhale completely to release any leftover tension. Gently let your breathing return to normal and let your whole body enjoy this time to relax.

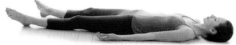

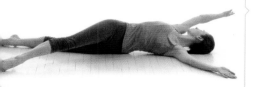

» their sleep improved that night. In 2005, Indian researchers put insomnia patients on a yoga program. After 6 months, the patients reported that it took less time to fall asleep, they slept longer, and they felt more rested.

I've had problems getting to sleep in the past and occasionally still do when I'm not doing enough yoga. Having a regular yoga practice rids you of unnecessary energy and keeps tension from hanging around in your body and mind. Practice this routine three times a week, on your mat or even in your bed, so that when it's time to rest, you can really rest.

Memory

Don't you sometimes wish you could run a Google search on your own memory? If you constantly rack your brain for phone numbers or passwords, I have a solution: A regular yoga practice can jog your memory by calming your nervous system and enhancing concentration. A 2009 study published in the journal *BioPsychoSocial Medicine* found that a combination of yoga and meditation helped improve volunteers' ability to recall information as measured by a simple memory test.

To help improve your memory, I'm going to have you work on doing headstands. This sequence will »

Try this routine every day for 2 weeks in addition to your regular yoga practice and you will be on your way to mastering headstand. Stay at the stage that is challenging for you. You might be on the first pose for a week or more. That's OK. Your headstand will be easy when you are aligned and strong enough to hold it. Work on the preparation that will get you there. If you jump ahead, you will probably fall, get frustrated, and not build the base you need to be confident. Practicing yoga is about staying where you are right now. When you apply focus, effort, and patience, you will get where you want to go.

the **ROUTINE**

Try to hold each step in the sequence for 5 deep inhales and exhales.

Working toward Headstand

Headstand is often referred to as the king of yoga poses. Practicing headstand benefits the endocrine, circulatory, lymphatic, nervous, respiratory, digestive, and musculoskeletal systems. It also calms the brain and leaves you feeling revitalized and clear-headed.

■ **Headstand Prep,**
One Heel to Hip
p. 104

Try one leg, then the other.

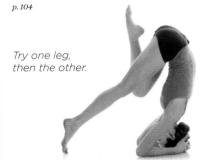

■ **Headstand Prep,**
Both Heels to Hips
p. 105

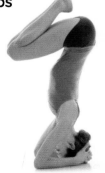

◼ Memory Meditation

After a vigorous practice, it's good to sit quietly for a few minutes and focus on your breath. Try this breath-focused meditation geared toward enhancing your memory:

Sit cross-legged with your hips up on a block and your knees resting out to the sides. Place your palms down on your thighs. Close your eyes and focus on your breath. If you have a thought, try to notice it without getting wrapped up in it. Send the thought on its way and return to your breath. Inhale through your nose for 4 counts. Hold the breath in for 4 counts. Exhale through your nose for 4 counts and hold the breath out for 4 counts. Repeat this breathing pattern for 2 minutes or 10 rounds, and then return to normal breathing. Continue to rest your attention on your breath for another 2 minutes, and then slowly open your eyes.

◼ Headstand Sock Slide
p. 103

Slide your feet back out to the extended position. Repeat this 20 times.

◼ Headstand Prep,
Feet Walked In
p. 104

◼ Headstand Prep
Leg Lift, Square Hips
p. 105

◼ Headstand
p. 106

» improve blood-flow through your brain cells, resulting in clearer and more powerful thinking. Don't get nervous if you haven't done a headstand since you were 5. We'll take this slowly and in stages. Yoga isn't just about nailing the pose. Maintaining a calm focus and ease of mind while moving through the poses is more important than achieving any final pose. If you are brand new to headstands, you should probably find a teacher who can guide you through the sequence in person. Also, using a wall for support is a good idea if you are a beginner.

Relaxation

Without rest, your body and mind can't decompress from the day. How often do you get sucked into thankless tasks like organizing receipts or folding clothes when you're trying to relax? The problem isn't those distractions (everyone has them!); it's your restless brain and body. If you haven't moved enough during the day, your brain tries to compensate by making your body feel restless so it can move. But these feelings can backfire and draw you into unnecessary tasks when you really need to simply relax. Do this sequence three times a week to engage your muscles and your mind so you can fully enjoy your chill-out time.

the ROUTINE *Try the following sequence, staying in each pose for 5 deep inhales and exhales.*

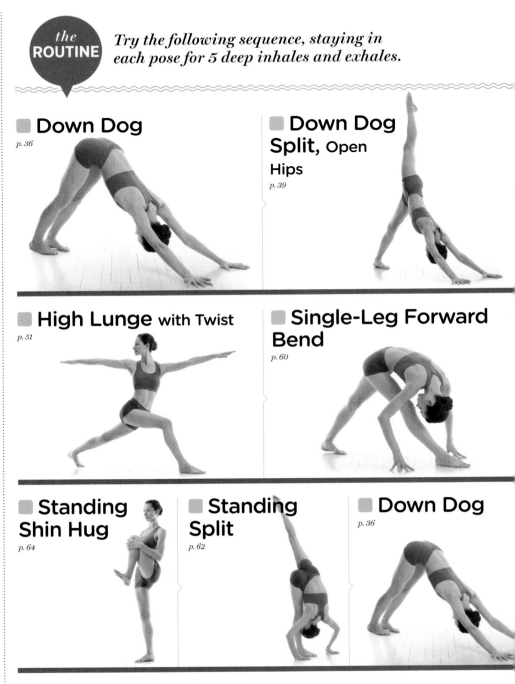

☐ Down Dog
p. 36

☐ Down Dog Split, Open Hips
p. 39

☐ High Lunge with Twist
p. 51

☐ Single-Leg Forward Bend
p. 60

☐ Standing Shin Hug
p. 64

☐ Standing Split
p. 62

☐ Down Dog
p. 36

Low Lunge
p. 46

High Lunge
p. 50

Warrior 3, Hands on Shin
p. 55

Half Moon
p. 66

Child's Pose
p. 92

Now repeat this routine once on the other side and you'll be really ready to chill out!

TAKE IT FROM
Tara

CLUTTER-FREE AND CALM

Make your bed. I have a hard time with this one, but this is advice I should take myself, and making the bed is just the beginning. Having clutter all over the house, dishes in the sink, clothes on the floor, and the bed unmade adds up to chaos in the mind and body. Try it for a week: Pick up after yourself. Clean the dishes after each meal. Put away your papers after you work. Make your bed in the morning. If you already do these simple tasks, you surely know the benefits of a peaceful home. Making your home peaceful by picking up after yourself is part of your yoga practice. Your life carries onto your mat and the other way around, too.

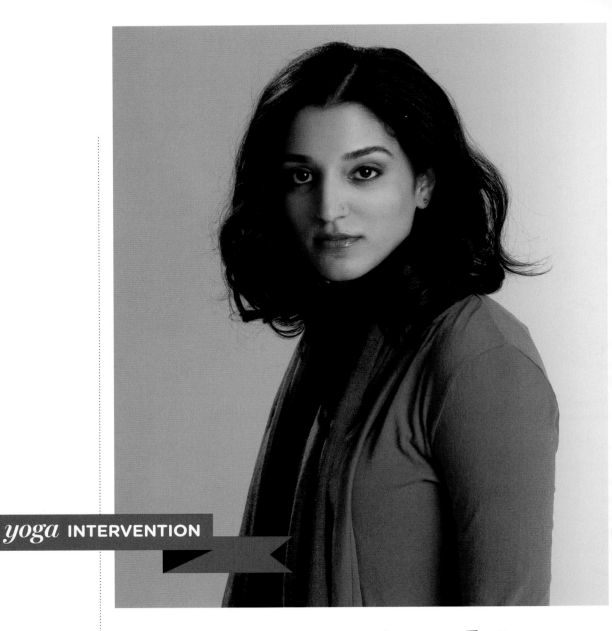

Namrata Tripathi

THE ISSUE: STRESS MANAGEMENT AND SLEEP PROBLEMS

*"I love the squat hang pose (page 35) because it melts away tension.
And I love warrior 2 (page 53) because it helps me reenergize."*

With a heavy workload as an executive editor at a major publishing house in New York City and a busy life outside the office, 30-year-old Namrata (Nami, for short) often forgets to slow down and take time for herself.

Even sleep gets short shrift. "I'll get 7 hours, but only on a rare good night. It's usually a lot less than that. And I've never found anything that has helped," she says.

In the past, Nami considered trying yoga but "found it challenging to find the right class, teacher, and studio that made me feel at home," she says. Then, in early 2009, a friend dragged her to Strala, and she never looked back.

"All of a sudden I could sleep," Nami says, describing the night of her first yoga class. "I went home and zonked out for 11 hours straight! I actually started worrying that yoga was going to put me into a sleep coma. My schedule won't allow for that."

When you practice yoga, your body begins to learn what it needs. In Nami's case, it was instant and dramatic. She needed sleep. Fair warning: The needs of your body are sometimes different from the wants of your mind. Yoga practice fuses the two, calming the mind and channeling behavior along the right path for optimal health.

"After I started practicing yoga more regularly, my sleep schedule started to level off at an acceptable 7 to 8 hours," Nami says. "I feel more rested and refreshed in the morning now than before I started doing yoga."

Nami also discovered a key to heading off work stress: scheduling a class immediately after work to create a boundary between her job and the rest of her life. "It resets my mind," she says. "I feel calmer when I get home. Otherwise I wouldn't be able to settle down, and my mind would be racing."

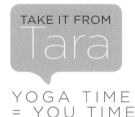

TAKE IT FROM
Tara

YOGA TIME = YOU TIME

Often we create our own stress. We pack our schedules so full that we don't even have room to breathe. When you practice yoga, not only does it give you that hour on the mat to feel calm and refreshed, it also gives you insight into and perspective on how you're living your life.

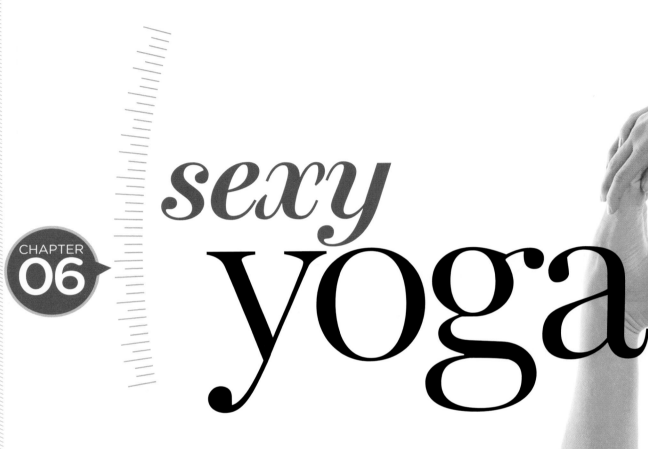

sexy
yoga

Radiate sexiness with routines
that take you from mat to bed

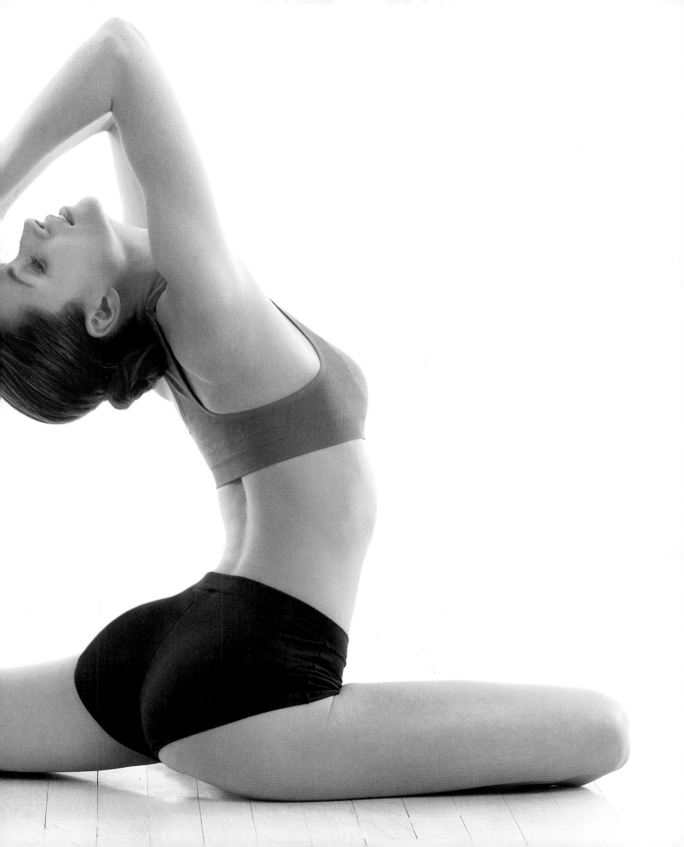

One

unmistakable thing you'll notice after starting to practice yoga is that it puts you in intimate touch with your breath, body, and mind. The natural outcome is a heightened awareness of your feelings—both emotional and physical. Ask anyone who's into yoga and they can probably describe (at a level of detail bordering on TMI) what's going on with their body at any given time. You may not want to know every last thing about their bodily functions, but it doesn't hurt to be aware of yours, if for no other reason than it could make your sex life a whole lot better.

In an experiment at the University of Texas at Austin, researchers created a situation in which women with low body image were made aware of their bodies by placing electrodes on their own skin while standing nude in front of a mirror. The scientists then asked them to sit and listen to an erotic audiotape. (Meanwhile, they asked another group of women to listen to the tape but skip the body-viewing step.) Afterward, the women who'd done the mirror exercise reported higher levels of arousal than the others. The scientists believe that being consciously aware of your body can enhance how you perceive erotic messages and make them more powerful.

You don't have to stand naked in front of a mirror to benefit from the kind of body awareness yoga can give you. All it takes is a committed practice and time on the mat. And body awareness isn't the only thing you'll walk away with. Yoga, like any other form of physical exercise, increases bloodflow throughout your entire body, including to your pleasure centers. Major bonus.

Practicing yoga also teaches you how to be mindful. I talked about mindfulness earlier in the book, but to review: Mindfulness is a term often used to describe a peaceful state of mental clarity in which smart decisions and good choices become crystal clear. Apart from all the fabulous body benefits of yoga, mindfulness is probably the greatest gift yoga will give you, because it

spills over into so many parts of your life. You learn to make healthy food choices, for example, or sensible relationship decisions. You feel calmer about those choices, and your confidence and well-being go way up.

For years, psychologists have used mindfulness techniques with patients who have mental and physical illnesses, and now sex therapists are starting to use them to treat sexual arousal disorders. In a 2008 study published in the *Journal of Sexual Medicine*, a group of female subjects participated in three mindfulness education seminars and viewed an erotic film before and after each one. The women reported significantly lower levels of desire after watching the flick before mindfulness training than they did when they saw it after the class.

Sexual hang-ups and intimacy and desire issues can arise from unhealthy practices and attitudes about life. As a discipline, yoga helps you tune in to healthy attitudes that make you feel good. The better you feel, the sexier you are. The sexier you are, the more open you are to your sensuality. The more open you are to your sensuality, well, the better you feel. Think of it as a pleasure cycle—and enjoy every minute of it.

Arousal and Desire

I recently read this statistic: Twenty-six percent of American women report having trouble becoming aroused during sex. And in a survey published in the *Archives of Internal Medicine*, more than one in three women admitted to experiencing low sexual desire in the past month. Hello—that's more than 40 million of us! Talk about frustrating.

Unfortunately it doesn't surprise me.

Guys seem to have it pretty easy when it comes to sexual arousal: They get turned on. Brain shuts down. Enjoyment ensues. For most women, it's more complex. To feel even the slightest bit of desire, our head has to be in the game. A 2003 study at Northwestern University found that even when women show the physical signs of sexual excitement below the belt, if they're not mentally turned on they won't feel a thing.

Getting in the mood often is hindered by stress and anxiety. It's hard to feel sexy when you're worried about your to-do list, or when your mind is racing. Your yoga practice can help you put things in perspective (hello, mindfulness!), so you can push aside distractions and feel in the moment and excited.

Done twice a week, this routine focuses on reducing tension in the body and mind and building sensual energy.

the **ROUTINE**

Try the following sequence, staying in each pose for 5 deep inhales and exhales, unless otherwise noted.

Up Dog
p. 131

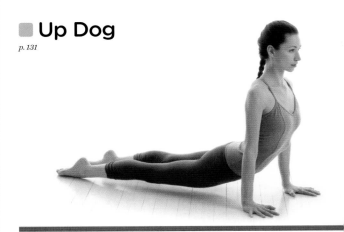

Supported Bridge
on One Block
p. 135

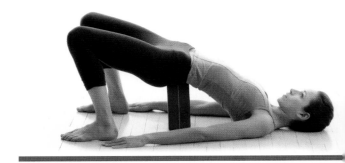

■ Bow

p. 131

Stay here for 10 long, deep breaths, then slowly lower your arms and legs so you're resting on your belly. Rest your arms along your sides. Turn the left side of your face to the mat and relax for 5 long, deep breaths. Repeat.

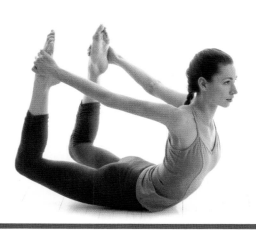

■ Seated Easy Twist

p. 73

Twist to one side, then the other.

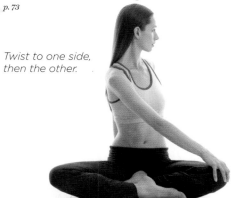

Bonding with Your Partner

Even if you're in a class, yoga can feel like a solitary endeavor. Half the time you have your eyes closed! So it's nice to have a reason to practice with your partner. If yoga is important to you, sharing it with your partner lets him in on a key part of your life and helps you feel closer to one another. Supporting each other in various poses builds trust and communication. And it's kind of like foreplay—you're breathing together, sweating together, and moving together. Try this sequence once a week to get in tune with yourself and your partner. (Make sure to switch roles each time so you both get the benefits!) It will reduce »

the ROUTINE

Try the following sequence, staying in each pose for 5 deep inhales and exhales, unless otherwise noted.

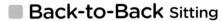

▪ Back-to-Back Sitting
p. 136

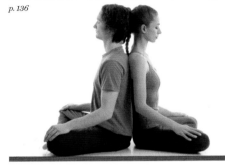

▪ Back-to-Back Lean
p. 138

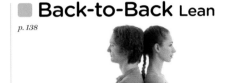

▪ Seated Straddle
p. 140

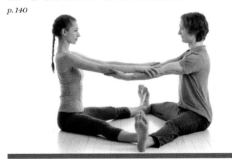

▪ Forward Bend
Back Press
p. 141

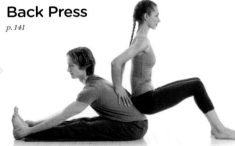

▪ Corpse
Partner Adjustment
p. 142

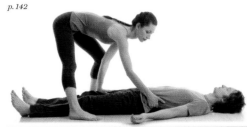

▪ Corpse
Neck Massage
p. 143

Continue for a few deep breaths.

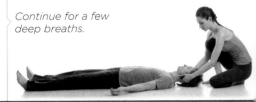

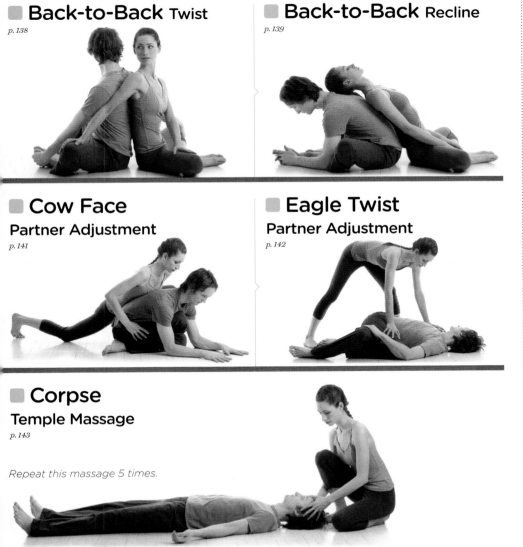

Back-to-Back Twist
p. 138

Back-to-Back Recline
p. 139

Cow Face
Partner Adjustment
p. 141

Eagle Twist
Partner Adjustment
p. 142

Corpse
Temple Massage
p. 143

Repeat this massage 5 times.

» stress levels, make communication easier, and heighten your intuition, all of which lead to a deeper level of intimacy.

Don't be surprised if you end up heading straight to the bedroom when you're finished.

Orgasm

All that breathing

and staying in the moment feels great, but there is another exciting payout from practicing yoga: more-satisfying orgasms. Recent research published in the *Journal of Sexual Medicine* looked at the effect of yoga on women's sexual function, including such factors as desire, arousal, lubrication, orgasm, and overall satisfaction. Among women under 45, the factor that improved the most after they participated in a 12-week yoga program was the quality of their orgasms. The researchers haven't pinpointed the exact reason for the improvement, but they suggest that any number of yoga's proven benefits—such as improved muscle tone in the pelvic region and stress reduction—are at work.

Whether you already climax easily or struggle to get there, a regular yoga practice relieves your body and brain of excess tension that may be holding you back from attaining some of the best pleasures of your life. Try this sequence twice a week to release tension in your hips, hamstrings, lower back, and brain. This will help to keep you in the moment and ready to experience and enjoy orgasms.

the **ROUTINE**

Try the following sequence, staying in each pose for 10 deep inhales and exhales.

Cow Face
p. 88

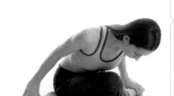

Ankle to Knee
p. 88

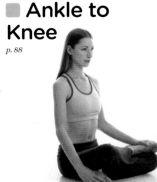

Split
with Block under Hip
p. 90

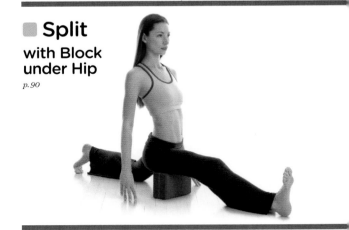

Compass Prep

p. 89

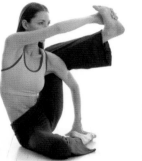

Compass

p. 89

Do the full compass pose only if you have no tension in compass prep and you'd like to go further.

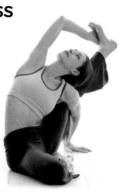

Reclining Goddess

p. 121

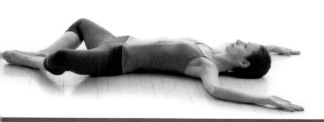

Repeat the whole sequence on the other side.

TAKE IT FROM

Tara

HIPS DON'T LIE

Sexual and emotional tension is often stored in the hips. It's not uncommon for powerful feelings to rise up when working on deep hip openers, like the poses on this page. Stay in the moment with whatever is going on in your body and mind; it will help you both on the mat and in the bedroom.

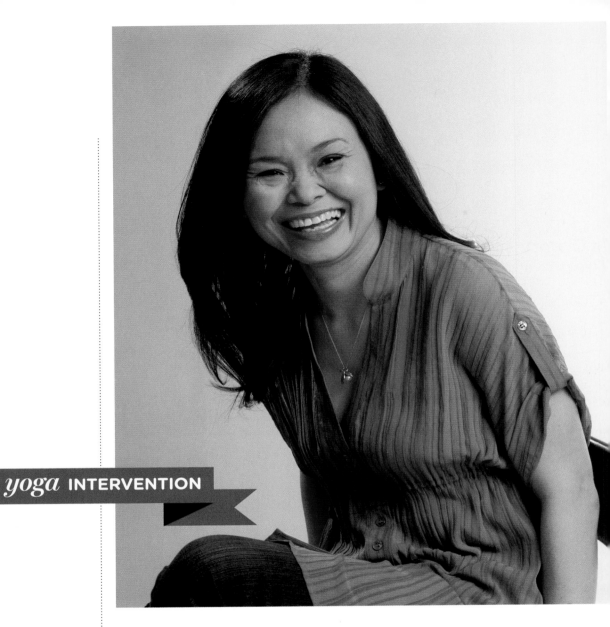

Liezl Panlilio

THE ISSUE: A LACKLUSTER SEX LIFE

"Practice pigeon pose. The hips carry a lot of tension, both physically and psychologically, and after spending a few long, deep breaths in pigeon (see page 90), I feel relaxed, open, and sexier."

After Liezl and her husband got married in 2000, they enjoyed all the perks of newlywed life, including lots of between-the-sheets fun.

But after they had their daughter in 2001, everything changed. "After Yssa was born, I felt self-conscious about my body, and my sex drive definitely suffered," says the 38-year-old graduate student.

When Liezl took her first yoga class at Strala in the summer of 2008, she wasn't looking to "fix" her sex life. After hearing so much about yoga's mind and body benefits, she "was just curious to try it," she says. But she was hooked after the first class. "I loved how it made me feel refreshed and open," she says. "It was different from any other kind of physical activity I tried." She has been a regular ever since.

After 2 months of coming to class regularly, Liezl noticed an unexpected perk: She felt sexier.

"Yoga was making me more comfortable in my body," she says. Learning to hold poses and control her breathing led to a pretty amazing physical transformation, and Liezl's insecurities were eventually replaced with confidence. "I feel fantastic about my body now," she says. The bonus? "I get aroused more easily, and I'm more relaxed."

She also enjoyed a newfound enthusiasm for experimenting in bed with positions she never would have imagined trying before. "It helps that I'm a lot more flexible," she admits. Yoga also has helped Liezl be more aware of her breath and body and let go of mental distractions, which helps her relax and enjoy sex. She's more focused in everything she does, on and off the mat.

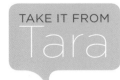

TAKE IT FROM
Tara

INTIMATE BREATHS

Holding your breath tenses your body and mind and brings you out of the moment, in your everyday life and in the bedroom. The next time you're getting intimate, focus on guiding your attention back to your breath; you'll be giving yourself the gift of living in the moment, which leads straight to fireworks in the sack. Trust me. It works.

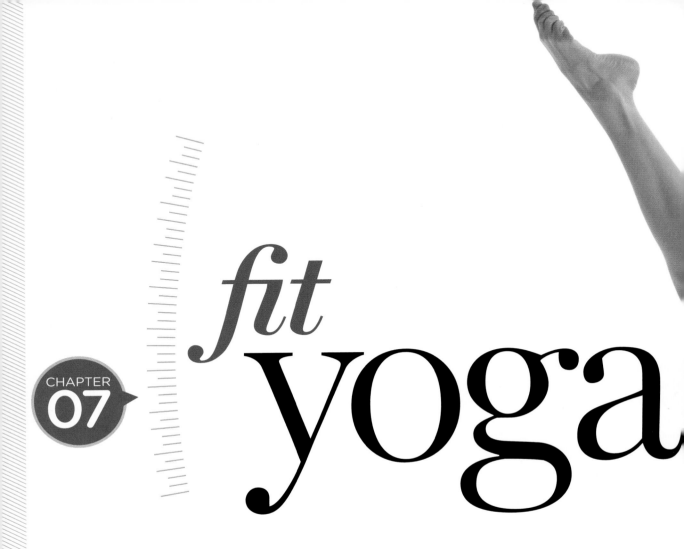

fit yoga

Sculpt a sexy yoga body
with poses that blast fat
and tone muscle

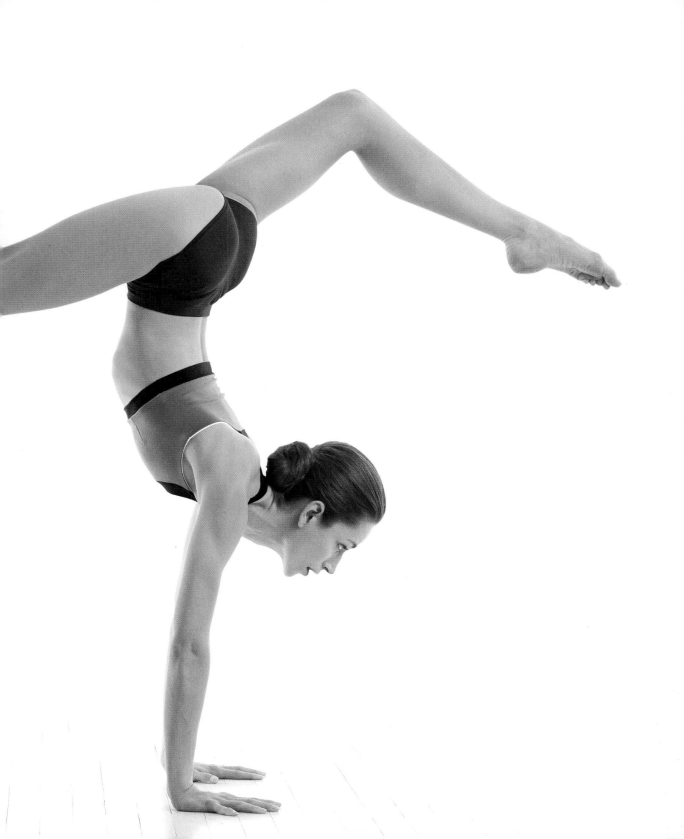

You need a healthy and fit body and mind to feel good and perform your best in any aspect of your life. Whether you're an athlete or a gym rat, or you just want to get the groceries home without throwing your back out, a consistent yoga practice can help. Here's what yoga does to make you fit:

■ Hones your balance . . . so your body can move with grace and efficiency.
■ Improves your flexibility . . . making you less susceptible to injury.
■ Increases your muscle stamina . . . so you can feel better all day long or train for that 5K you've been eyeing.
■ Builds your strength . . . giving you enviable muscle tone.
And all these qualities will make you better at any physical endeavor while preventing injury and speeding recovery.

   Here are some of the proven ways practicing yoga improves fitness. In a study published in the *Journal of Strength and Conditioning Research*, healthy young adults were divided into two groups. One followed an 8-week yoga program; the other did not.

At the end of the study period, only the yoga group gained leg strength, muscle control, and balance.

In a 2010 study at the City University of New York, researchers looked at the effect of yoga on functional fitness. (That's a buzzy term for workouts that train your body for everyday activities.) The study subjects were a group of 108 firefighters who took part in yoga classes at their station houses. Before and after the 6-week study period, they were tested on stability, mobility, and flexibility (things that measure functional fitness). What did the researchers find? Scores shot up significantly after the yoga, and more than half of the firefighters said their job performance improved.

Let's hope battling flames is more strenuous than anything you ever have to do. But if warrior poses and breathing exercises helped these guys perform better on the job, they're sure to help you—whether you sprint for a morning train, lug a toddler around all day, or stand on your feet for an entire night shift.

Those are pretty fantastic fitness benefits, if you ask me. But if you're looking to improve your 5K time, don't rely solely on your yoga practice. A few years ago, the American Council on Exercise gathered a group of healthy women who hadn't exercised or done yoga for 6 months. They were split into two groups: One group did nothing; the other did mellow hatha yoga for 55 minutes three times a week for 8 weeks. The yoga boosted strength, flexibility, endurance, and balance, though it didn't raise maximum heart rate or VO_2 max (the amount of oxygen a body converts into energy during each minute of maxed-out exercise—the higher the number, the fitter your lungs). There's no getting around it: Mellow styles of yoga generally aren't intense enough to push your heart rate superhigh. You're more likely to do that with more vigorous activities, like running or biking. But you'll perform any intense exercise more efficiently if you also practice yoga. In one study, athletes who regularly practiced pranayama, the kind of controlled breathing you do in yoga, were able to work harder and use less oxygen compared with athletes in a control group.

By focusing on four pillars of fitness—balance, flexibility, stamina, and strength—the following routines will give you more energy, improve your overall fitness, and leave you with a sleek, sculpted body.

Balance

Working on balance poses helps with focus, speed, control, and injury prevention whether you are a professional athlete, a weekend warrior, or simply someone who feels like she's walking a tightrope all day. Developing balance trains your whole body to work effectively as a unit. This helps to develop your muscles evenly and prevents injuries by putting all your parts in tune with each other. It also eases your mind. When you feel balanced in your body, you have a better chance of feeling balanced in your mind. One is a reflection of the other. Practice this routine twice a week for the best results.

the **ROUTINE**

Try the following sequence, staying in each pose for 5 deep inhales and exhales.

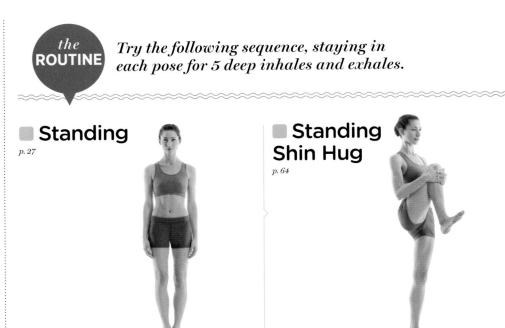

Standing
p. 27

Standing Shin Hug
p. 64

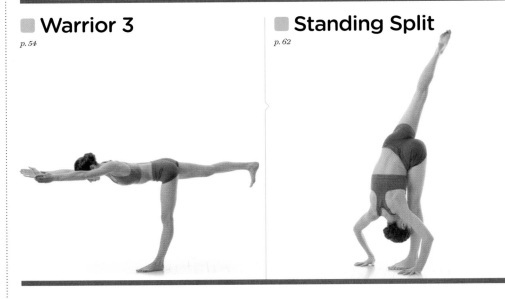

Warrior 3
p. 54

Standing Split
p. 62

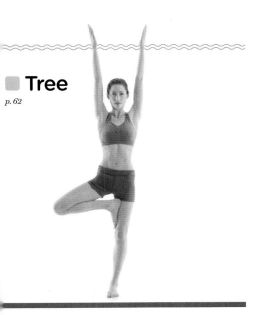

Tree

p. 62

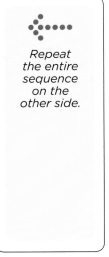

Repeat the entire sequence on the other side.

TAKE IT FROM
Tara

STAY IN THE GAME

Many trainers and coaches include yoga in their training plans. Why? Because it's effective at preventing and relieving chronic injuries and reducing postworkout soreness. A study in the Journal of Strength and Conditioning Research investigated whether women who practiced yoga had milder postworkout soreness. The answer was a definitive yes. Because of yoga's ability to stabilize the joints by strengthening the muscles around them, the concept of yoga therapy is catching on in the United States, where practitioners use yoga to treat patients recovering from sports injuries, surgery, and chronic pain. Patients get one-on-one attention with targeted poses, much as they would with traditional physical therapy. As for yoga helping you bounce back from an injury, there is compelling evidence that it can help relieve chronic conditions like carpal tunnel syndrome, arthritis, and back pain; not so much when it comes to, say, healing a sprained ankle, though.

I work with a lot of runners, a group in desperate need of yoga. Tight hamstrings, tight hips, and injuries are the natural results of constant pavement pounding. The most common reason I hear from runners for not embracing yoga is that they just don't have time. That's no excuse! You need no more than 15 minutes of yoga to reconnect your body with your breath, release tension in tight muscle groups, and focus your mind. And the advantages are too good to ignore: reduced injuries and faster recovery times.

Flexibility

Any time you fight stiff muscles, you waste energy. If you loosen up those muscles, you reduce that resistance so you can channel your energy to what you really want out of a workout: calorie annihilation—and the sexy body that results.

Flexibility takes breath, time, and patience. Each time you exhale, it's an opportunity to release tension in your body. If you hold your breath, you hold on to tension, and there's a good chance you'll strain a muscle.

You also need to spend time in each pose. Your muscles need time to open up. Try this routine three times a week (with patience), and you will see and feel dramatic results.

the
ROUTINE

Try the following sequence, staying in each pose for 10 deep inhales and exhales.

Low Lunge
p. 46

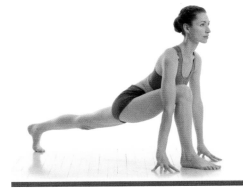

Low Lunge, Sit on Back Heel, Forward Bend
p. 50

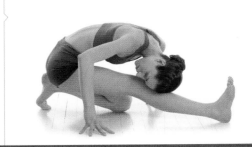

Split with Two Blocks
p. 91

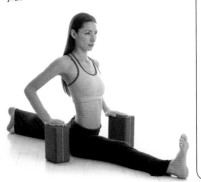

Repeat the previous sequence on the other side, then move on to the following poses.

Seated Wide Leg Straddle
p. 77

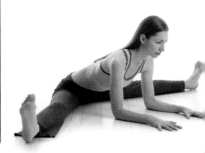

■ Single-Leg Forward Bend
p. 60

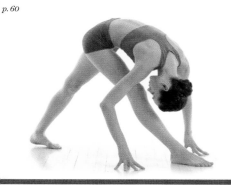

■ Pigeon
p. 90

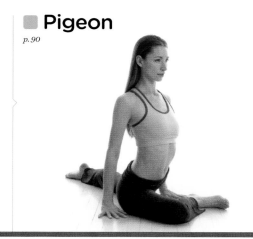

■ Seated Wide Leg Straddle **with Twist**
p. 78

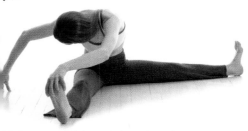

Twist to one side and then the other. Carefully walk your fingertips forward. Place your forearms on the floor and reach your chest forward and your hips back.

■ Seated Forward Bend
p. 74

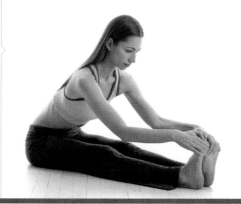

There is a common misconception that flexibility is a direct result of stretching. Yet just hearing the word stretching can make your body and mind clench. The truth is, flexibility comes from releasing tension. Yoga teaches you how to breathe deeply in each pose, which releases tension in tight areas of your body. I encourage you to shift your thinking from stretching a muscle, which leads to tension and injury, to releasing tension through breathing. Think of each exhale as an opportunity to release tension and each inhale as a way to lengthen and fill your body with oxygen.

Stamina

When your chest, ribs, and back are tight, every breath takes more energy than it would if those areas were open and relaxed. And when your whole body is tight, every movement re-quires more effort. When it comes to performance and everyday exis-tence, you need every ounce of energy you can get. Stamina improves when your body is open.

In order to main-tain a good fitness level, it's impor-tant to challenge your body. If you practice the same routine for a long period of time, your body will get used to it and your results will plateau. You probably don't want to eat the same thing for dinner every »

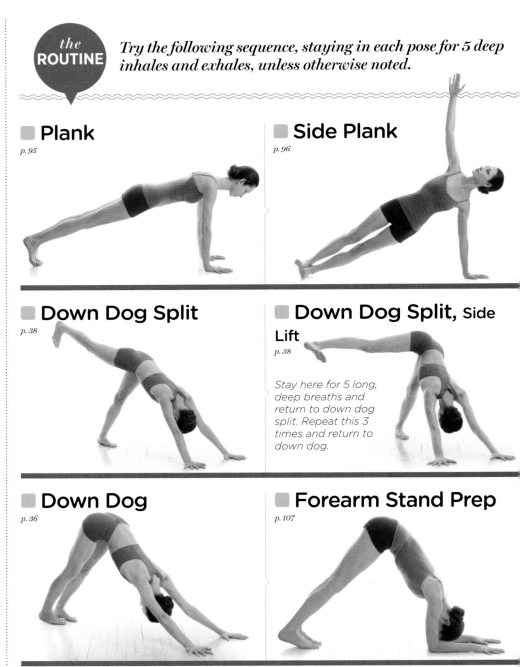

the ROUTINE

Try the following sequence, staying in each pose for 5 deep inhales and exhales, unless otherwise noted.

▢ Plank
p. 95

▢ Side Plank
p. 96

▢ Down Dog Split
p. 38

▢ Down Dog Split, Side Lift
p. 38

Stay here for 5 long, deep breaths and return to down dog split. Repeat this 3 times and return to down dog.

▢ Down Dog
p. 36

▢ Forearm Stand Prep
p. 107

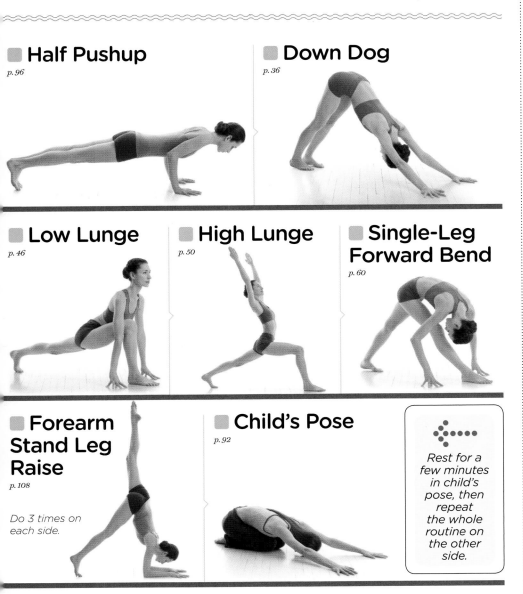

Half Pushup
p. 96

Down Dog
p. 36

Low Lunge
p. 46

High Lunge
p. 50

Single-Leg Forward Bend
p. 60

Forearm Stand Leg Raise
p. 108

Do 3 times on each side.

Child's Pose
p. 92

Rest for a few minutes in child's pose, then repeat the whole routine on the other side.

» night, and your body doesn't do its best with the same fitness routine, either. You can tailor your yoga routines to help with and achieve a wide variety of goals. Challenge yourself twice a week with this sequence to improve your stamina and boost your overall strength, tolerance, and willpower.

Strength

Regardless of whether you have athletic ambitions, strength is essential for getting you through your busy day. Imagine hailing a cab or hoisting your carry-on bag into an overhead compartment if you couldn't lift your arms. These actions take muscle. I'm not saying you need bodybuilder bulk, but you do need some power. And along with muscle comes a sculpted "notice me!" body.

When it comes to getting stronger without getting hurt, you want to create a balance between strength and flexibility so your muscles develop a full range of motion. Unlike most traditional or sport-specific workouts, which emphasize a particular set of muscle groups, yoga cultivates balanced strength, carving out a capable body that endures more work with less effort. How? By requiring your entire body to work as a whole, which strengthens weaker muscle groups and trains stronger muscle groups at the same time.

Balance in the body is great for performance, but yoga also gives you a mental edge by teaching you to maintain a clear, calm, and focused mind in easy and stressful situations alike is a useful side effect of practice. For best results, do this sequence three times a week.

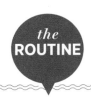

the ROUTINE

Try the following sequence, staying in each pose for 5 deep inhales and exhales.

Plank
p. 95

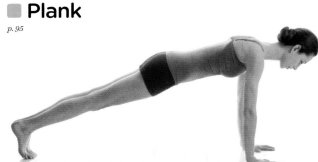

Knee to Forehead
p. 101

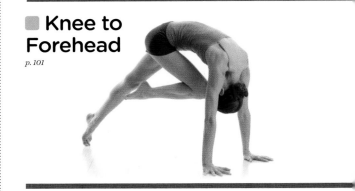

Warrior 3
p. 54

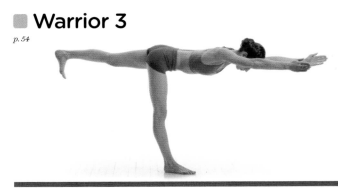

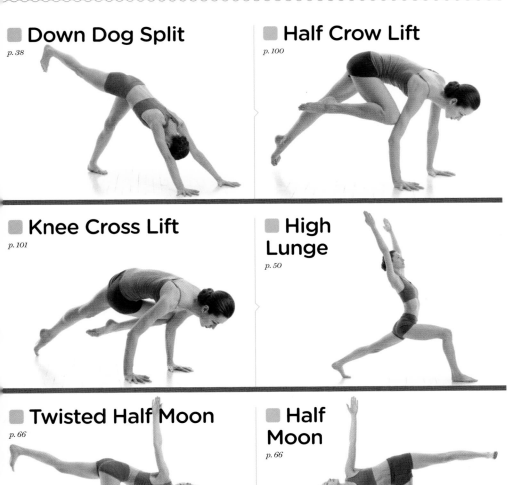

■ Down Dog Split
p. 38

■ Half Crow Lift
p. 100

■ Knee Cross Lift
p. 101

■ High Lunge
p. 50

■ Twisted Half Moon
p. 66

■ Half Moon
p. 66

continued

Strength (continued)

the ROUTINE

Stay in each pose for 5 deep inhales and exhales.

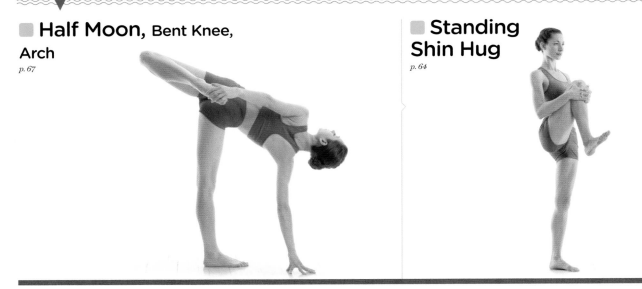

◻ **Half Moon,** Bent Knee, Arch
p. 67

◻ **Standing Shin Hug**
p. 64

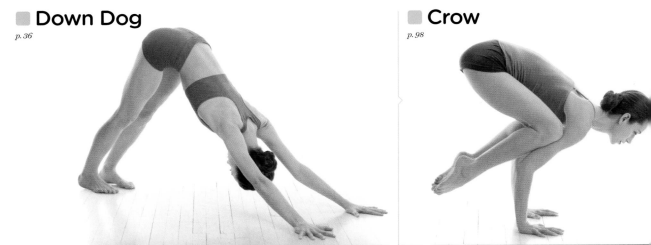

◻ **Down Dog**
p. 36

◻ **Crow**
p. 98

Tree
p. 62

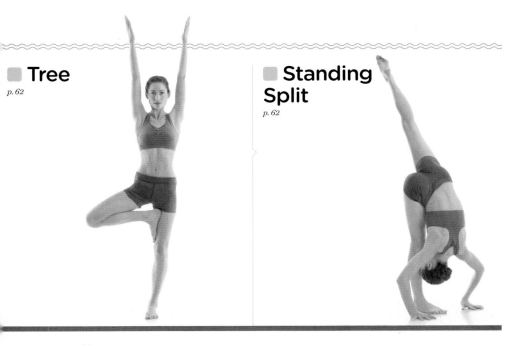

Standing Split
p. 62

Standing Forward Bend, Calf Hold
p. 32

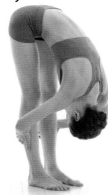

Repeat the entire sequence on the other side.

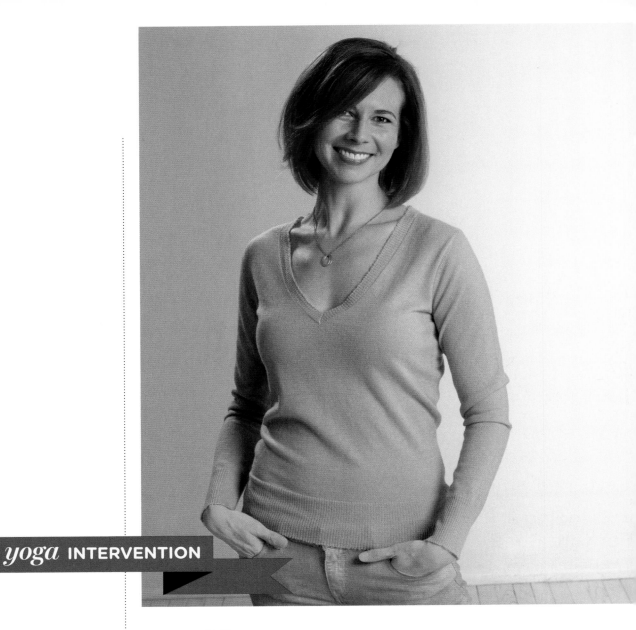

Tiffany West

THE ISSUE: SPORTS INJURIES

"Own your practice. The instructor will give you a series of poses, but you're under no obligation to do them. If you have an injury, tell the teacher before class starts, and he or she will usually suggest a variation that should work better for you. Don't feel that you have to do what the teacher says if it doesn't feel right."

As a lifelong athlete, 33-year-old Tiffany West has a fierce competitive spirit. It was helpful on the lacrosse field and in the boat she crewed for her high school rowing team.

Not so much when it forced her to push so hard she wound up injured multiple times, though. "After five foot surgeries, a torn meniscus in each knee, and most recently a herniated disk, I'm pretty limited in the kinds of exercise I can do," says Tiffany, a global leadership fellow at the World Economic Forum.

Each stint on the sidelines took an emotional toll. "I was always afraid of losing all my fitness," she says. So 8 years ago she turned to yoga to stay in shape—and off the injured list. At first it was hard to ditch the athlete's mindset. "I had to let go of certain desires ('I will do a headstand no matter what')," she says. But eventually her no-pain-no-gain attitude began to soften. "Practicing yoga helped me focus just on myself, rather than on a competitor," she says. "I'm less hard on myself when I'm on the mat than I ever was in sports. Knees feeling especially creaky today? I back off so they're not strained. Lower back can't handle plow pose right now? I'll try a new pose or a variation instead."

For Tiffany, yoga has been the key to finding a healthy balance between challenging herself physically and staying injury-free. "My injuries forced me to reexamine how I view the world, and yoga helped me go from 'win at all costs' to a new goal: 'Enjoy, explore, and learn.'"

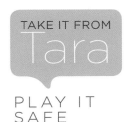

TAKE IT FROM
Tara

PLAY IT
SAFE

If you've been injured, be sure to see a doctor before starting yoga. You really don't want to push, pull, or bend your body in a way that could aggravate sensitive areas.

gorgeous yoga

Moves that get your glow on

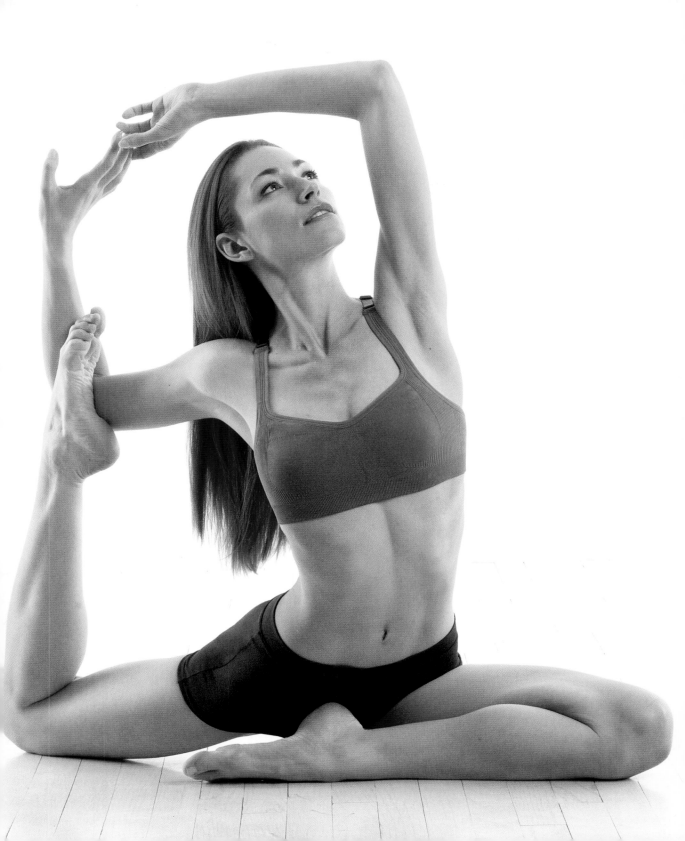

If

If you've adopted any of the techniques from previous chapters, you've probably discovered a new sense of calm and confidence. You're less fatigued. You stand taller. You hold your head up high. You suck in your belly. Maybe you've even noticed your skin has a little more glow to it and you smile more easily.

No matter what facial features or body you were born with, when you feel good, you look good. And practicing yoga and meditation, well, they make you feel amazing.

It doesn't hurt that science backs up the body-mind-beauty connection. We've already established that yoga and meditation are all-star stress-soothers. But what you might not know is that your mind (and by association, stress) is closely connected to the largest organ in your body—your skin. Ever blush? I thought so. That's just one example of how what you're feeling on the inside can show on the outside.

It makes sense, and here's why: Your skin contains an intricate web of tiny nerve endings that relays messages to and from your brain. Your skin also houses an army of immune system cells that fight bacterial and viral invaders. Imagine your skin as a Gore-Tex raincoat—an impermeable layer that swaddles your flesh, bones, and organs, and regulates how your body responds to environmental influences such as heat, cold, and even pollution. When your nerves are out of whack—you're stressed or bummed out—it interferes with your skin's protective powers, making it more susceptible to pain and infection, the way a torn raincoat lets in water. In one study at Cornell University's Weill Medical College, scientists subjected volunteers to psychologically stressful situations and then gave them each a microscopic skin wound. The outcome? The volunteers' skin took longer than usual to repair itself. Along those same lines, research links stress to a number of common skin problems, from acne to warts. Some doctors believe the connection is so strong that a new medical specialty called psychodermatology has emerged in recent years. These mainstream doctors at such respected institutions as Johns Hopkins and Harvard are using alternative techniques, including biofeedback, meditation, guided imagery, and yoga, to help treat a host of skin disorders.

I encourage you to think of your yoga practice as an approach to beauty that works from the inside out. Moving through the poses and monitoring your breath revitalizes your entire body from a cellular level. Once you become hooked on yoga as your beauty secret, you'll have no need for artificial and harmful gimmicks like harsh chemicals, needles, or surgery. And through the mindfulness you learn from practice, you'll naturally gravitate toward healthier eating and other practices that keep you looking good and feeling great.

Clear Skin

You'll usually break a sweat when you practice most athletic styles of yoga. Dripping sweat during down dog means that you're not only challenging your body, you're also torching calories and building strength. You are also doing good work to clear your pores, soften your skin, and rid your body of toxins. All you need to do is put in the effort on your mat to get the benefits. And don't worry about all that perspiration causing your skin to break out. A 2008 study found that exercise-induced sweating does not cause acne. Do this routine twice a week to start sweating your way to great skin.

the **ROUTINE**

Try the following sequence, staying in each pose for 5 deep inhales and exhales.

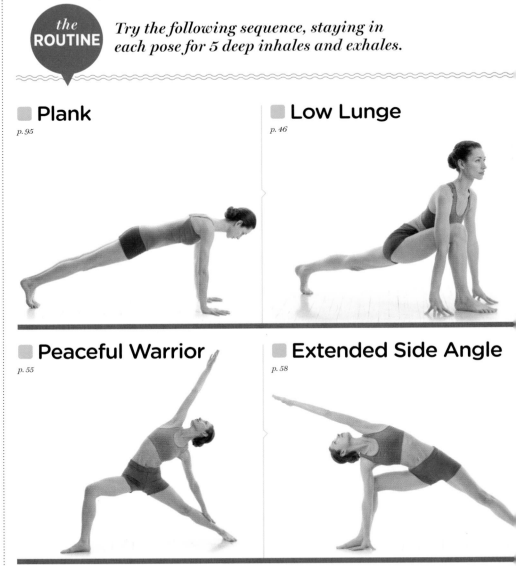

Plank
p. 95

Low Lunge
p. 46

Peaceful Warrior
p. 55

Extended Side Angle
p. 58

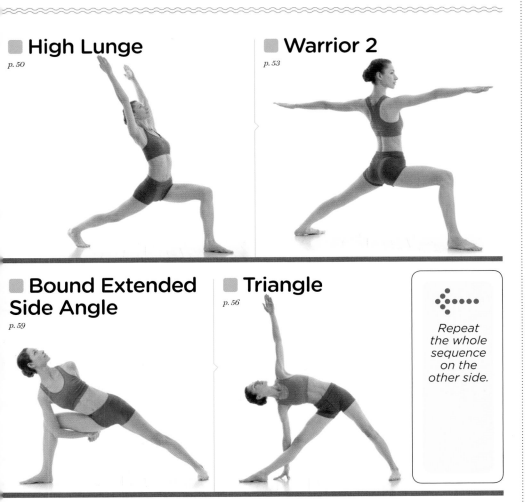

High Lunge
p. 50

Warrior 2
p. 53

Bound Extended Side Angle
p. 59

Triangle
p. 56

Repeat the whole sequence on the other side.

LISTEN TO YOUR BODY

We each have our own comfort zone. Pushing safely past it helps build strength and lets the sweat pour. Make sure you are working hard, but correctly and in alignment. You can always reach a little farther and extend a little more while listening to your body and breath to keep within your safe range. If your breath gets short and difficult, back off just enough to return it to long and deep. Relax your mind, and extend your body again when you're ready.

Confidence

A huge part of looking fresh and youthful is how you feel about yourself. When you're confident, you stand up straighter, smile more, and have more energy. A sure way to boost confidence off the mat is to work on poses you find intimidating. Even if you're already a whiz at challenging poses, in yoga there is always another one to master. These routines focus on moving into a back bend and working toward a handstand. We'll build slowly to each, so you can celebrate mini-accomplishments and gain confidence incrementally along the way. For best results, do this sequence three times a week.

the ROUTINE

Try the following sequence, staying in each pose for 20 deep inhales and exhales. At the dog split, begin holding the pose for 10 breaths.

☐ Sphinx
p. 130

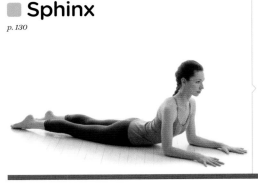

☐ Up Dog
p. 131

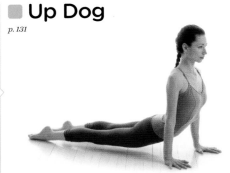

☐ Plank
p. 95

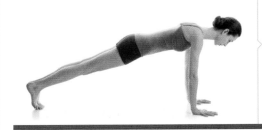

☐ Supported Bridge
on Two Blocks
p. 135

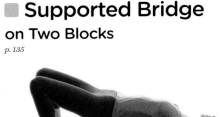

☐ Knee Hug
p. 121

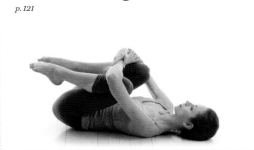

☐ Down Dog Split
p. 38

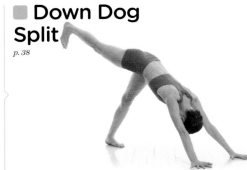

Child's Pose
p. 92

Down Dog
p. 36

Supported Bridge
on One Block
p. 135

Bridge, Hands Interlaced
p. 134

Handstand
at Wall
p. 109

Handstand
p. 110

TAKE IT FROM
Tara

WORKING
TOWARD A
HANDSTAND

Handstands take a lot of strength and perfect alignment, but are lots of fun to try and loads of fun when you master them. Practicing handstands also gives us a confidence boost and the ability to overcome fears.

Glowing Skin

In helping you manage stress, your yoga practice balances your hormones and boosts healthy bloodflow to your skin. This can help you get better sleep so you can say good-bye to eye bags and dark circles, allow- ing your skin to stay supple and smooth. And the muscle tone you gain from yoga practice also firms up your skin. Try this sequence twice a week to restore healthy bloodflow and bring your skin back to its natural state of gorgeous.

the **ROUTINE**

Try the following sequence, staying in each pose for 10 deep inhales and exhales, unless otherwise noted.

◼ Spine Roll
p. 83

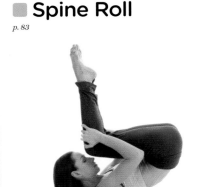

◼ Plow
p. 112

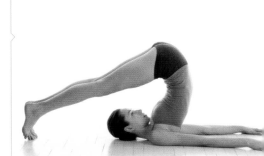

◼ Single Leg Extension
p. 125

Repeat the leg extension on the other side.

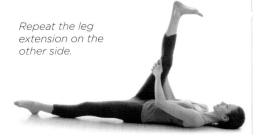

◼ Corpse
p. 126

After resting in corpse fo 10 breaths, carefully bend your knees to your chest and roll over onto your right side. Rest here for 5 long, deep inhales and exhales, then gently bring yourself up to sit.

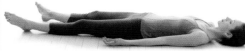

Shoulder Stand

p. 114

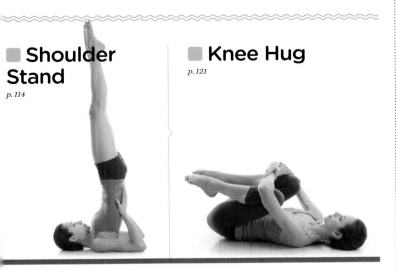

Knee Hug

p. 121

Seated Meditation

p. 69

Close your eyes and follow your breath. Stay here for 3 minutes.

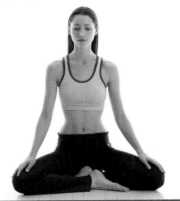

TAKE IT FROM

Tara

BUILDING AWARENESS

I was introduced to the formal practice of yoga in my teens, when vibrancy and aging were the last things on my mind. I delved more into the philosophy and meditative practices of yoga and didn't become interested in the physical advantages of the practice until a few years later, when my friends were worried about puffy eyes from partying all night.

My practice, for the most part, kept me out of the party scene (although I did have a little fun here and there). Clubs are filled with smoke, alcohol, and drugs that poison your body, and no one who keeps up that lifestyle looks or feels good for long. Life is more interesting when you're putting your efforts toward your interests and surrounding yourself with quality people. Yoga practice has a way of moving you away from destructive behaviors and optimizing how you use your time and life.

Eventually I realized that meditation, physical movement, and philosophy are not just interconnected; they're the same. A healthy mind and body are efficient tools for meditation, and every movement can be meditative. Yoga isn't a practice meant to take you out of your body. It is a practice to put you in touch with your body so you can experience life fully. By connecting you directly with everything you need to be healthy, yoga leaves you feeling good and looking gorgeous. There's nothing superficial about it. Your whole body will thank you.

Smooth Skin

stress and helps you become aware of tension in your body. How many times have you noticed your face clenching up when you're worried about something? Over time, that clenching can etch itself permanently on your face. (Yes, that's why they're called "worry lines.") Practice this sequence three times a week to calm your mind and reduce the stress that causes chronic tension in the face.

the ROUTINE

Try the following sequence, staying in each pose for 5 deep inhales and exhales, unless otherwise noted.

Low Lunge, Back Knee Down, Hands on Front Knee
p. 48

Low Lunge, Back Knee Down, Palm Press
p. 49

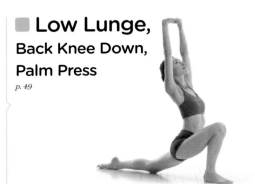

Single-Leg Forward Bend
p. 60

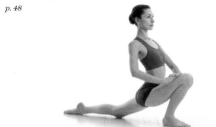

Warrior 3, Hands on Shin
p. 55

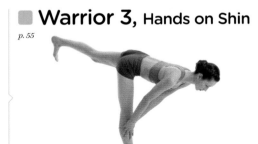

Forearm Stand Prep
p. 107

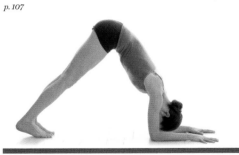

Plank Forearm
p. 97

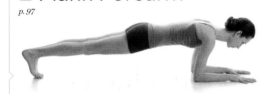

Stay here for 10 long, deep inhales and exhales, then press back to forearm stand prep. Move from forearm plank back to forearm stand prep 3 more times with the same breathing.

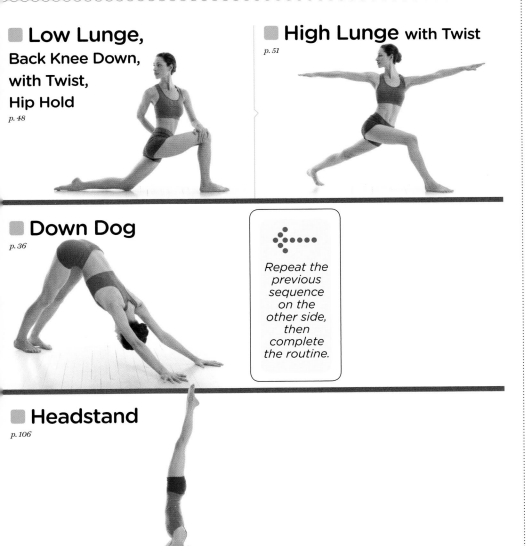

Low Lunge,
**Back Knee Down,
with Twist,
Hip Hold**
p. 48

High Lunge with Twist
p. 51

Down Dog
p. 36

Repeat the previous sequence on the other side, then complete the routine.

Headstand
p. 106

p. 48 · p. 51 · p. 36 · p. 106

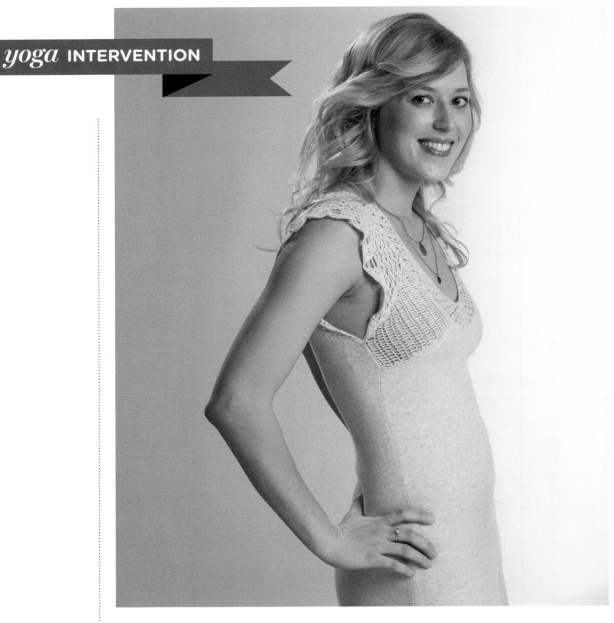

Verena Von Pfetten

THE ISSUE: LOW ENERGY LEVELS AND BAD SKIN

To get the most out of yoga, your body needs to be ready. "I discovered that the football-size Chipotle burrito that tasted so good at lunch did not taste so good in down dog pose later on," she says. Her yoga-friendly lunches now consist of healthier fare, like a salad with tons of good veggies.

As a busy Web site editor, 27-year-old Verena has a schedule full of deadlines, social obligations, and high-level stress—all of which combine to give her the (unwanted) gift of low energy and broken-out skin.

Even though she knew exercise could help her deal with stress, Verena always hated working out. "I tried the gym, even a personal trainer, and couldn't stick with it," she says. But after she started at Strala in August of 2008, her attitude changed. "The classes are challenging, but they're easier to stick with because we have fun," she says.

After a month or two of coming to class regularly, Verena noticed a visible change in the quality and tone of her skin. Her minor skin irritations and breakouts vanished, and her energy levels started to skyrocket. "Yoga makes me sleep like a baby," she says. "So the bags under my eyes need less and less concealer."

Verena also credits her newfound devotion to the yoga lifestyle with helping her eat more healthily and make all-around better decisions that affect her health—and, by association, how she looks. "I like going to class so much, I started scheduling my social life around it," she says. She goes to four or five classes a week, which leaves only one or two nights for social plans—which is a good thing: "I drink less, sleep more, and have a whole lot more time to myself."

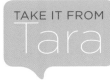

TAKE IT FROM
Tara

IT'S NEVER TOO EARLY

Verena is a great example of someone really understanding and achieving the benefits of yoga at a young age and making healthy lifestyle adjustments as a result. Why wait for your body to break down before you start to take care of it? Yoga can keep you looking good and feeling great your whole life, so it's best to start as early as you can.

healthy
yoga

Save your sick days with
health-focused routines

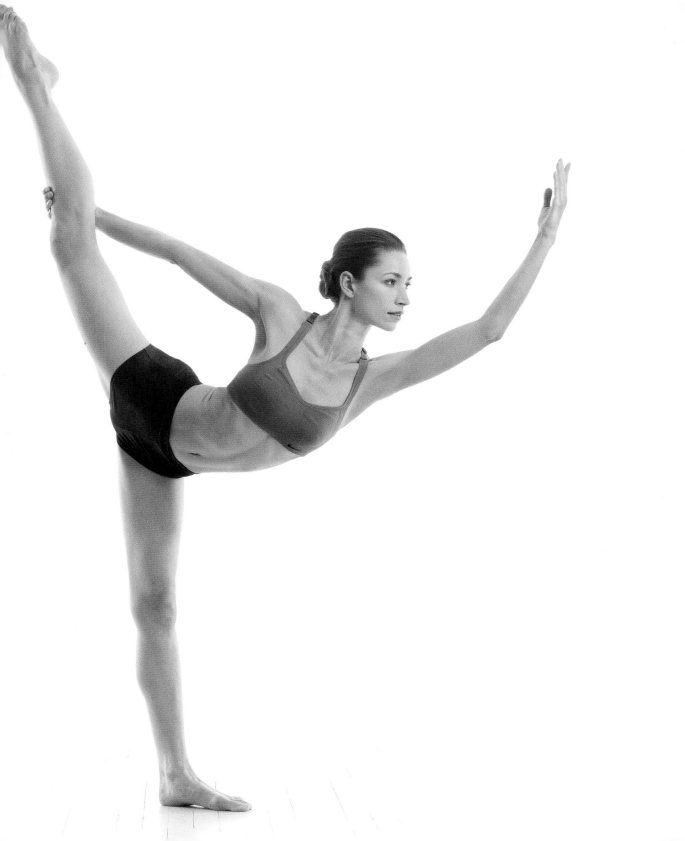

I want

you to pause for a moment and think about what it means to be healthy. Being healthy is about more than washing your hands after touching a doorknob or making sure you get a flu shot. It's bigger than taking a multivitamin, slathering on sunscreen, or visiting your gyno once a year.

Of course those things are absolutely important. But being healthy is also about simply feeling good on the inside. And feeling good on the inside leads to enjoying your life, achieving your goals, and looking good on the outside. Although good health is not glamorous in the same way as a slim body, a sexy attitude, or gorgeous skin is, without it, your chances of attaining any of those ideals plummet.

Thousands of years ago, yoga was developed as a system to improve and maintain health from the inside out. The ancient yogis in India fine-tuned it through years of trial and error using their intuition, powers of observation, and senses. Unlike in conventional Western medicine, the ancient yogis didn't believe a person was necessarily "healthy" if nothing appeared "wrong." Instead, you were truly healthy if every system in your body—from digestion to immunity to circulation—was functioning at its best. And that's precisely what they developed yoga to do: to optimize the body's everyday operations so that they're balanced and aligned—and can work the way they're intended to. The end result is a therapeutic practice that supports health and well-being by steadying and quieting the mind with meditation and breathing, combined with physical movements and poses.

Today, science is using its own language and methodology to explain the same benefits that ancient yogis observed. A recent search on the US National Library of Medicine databases yielded more than 1,300 scholarly articles on the subject of yoga. And the findings are worth every ounce of your attention. There is real evidence that yoga boosts immunity, improves mood, corrects imbalances that cause pain, and lowers blood sugar and blood pressure. There is compelling proof that it regulates hormones (including cortisol, the culprit in so many health issues from anxiety to weight gain), reduces disease-causing inflammation, even balances your circadian rhythms so you can get the rest you need to keep your body in top shape. These discoveries are exciting and offer solid hope for anyone who wants to lead a healthy lifestyle and sidestep serious illnesses like heart disease, diabetes and depression; for anyone who deals with pain on a regular basis; or for anyone who simply has an occasional run-in with a seasonal allergy or a hangover headache.

Great advances have come from scientific study, but it's not the only tool at your disposal. In fact, as the yogis discovered through thousands of years of experimentation, we have a full set of our own health tools already within us. You could say the proof is in the practice.

I encourage you to consider your regular yoga practice as a plan for maintaining total health. As the research in this chapter makes clear, it truly does have healing powers.

Allergies

Sixty-two percent of people with seasonal allergies say their runny noses, constant sneezing, and irritated sinuses make them, for lack of a better phrase, seriously miserable. The good news: Proven relaxation techniques such as yoga and meditation can help prevent or relieve those frustrating symptoms. Ohio State University researchers subjected a group of hay fever sufferers to stressful situations and then gave them allergy tests. When the subjects were the most stressed out, they had skin reactions that were twice as large as when they were calmer and the reactions lasted longer. According to the study, when stress hormones are elevated, it can weaken the immune system and prolong your allergic response. If you suffer from seasonal allergies, do this routine three times a week to clear your nasal passages, ease your stress levels, and restore balance to your system.

the **ROUTINE**

Try the following sequence, staying in each pose for 5 deep inhales and exhales, unless otherwise noted.

Calming Breath

Close your eyes, rest your palms on your thighs, and focus on your breath. If you start thinking about other things, guide your attention back to your breath. Breathe gently here for 1 minute.

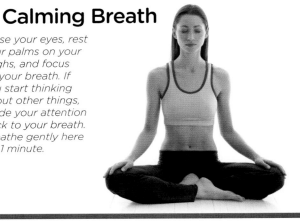

Standing Side Opener
p. 28

Do one side, then the other.

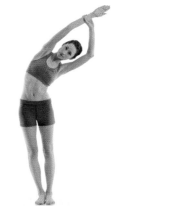

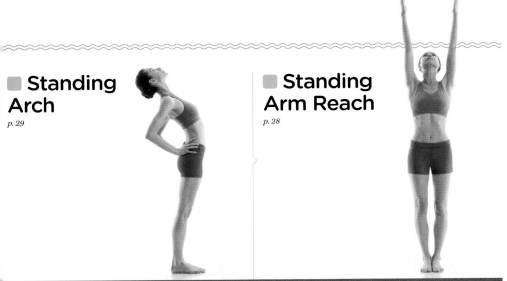

Standing
Arch
p. 29

Standing
Arm Reach
p. 28

Bellows Breathing
p. 14

Keep a tissue nearby. This exercise clears out the nasal passages, and you may need to wipe your nose.

Back Pain

More than 26 million

Americans between the ages of 20 and 64 have frequent back pain. And according to the National Institutes of Health, a sore back is the most common reason people under age 45 stop being active. Ask anyone with a "bad back" and they'll tell you it can make accomplishing even the simplest task much harder. But back pain doesn't have to be inevitable—a number of studies have shown a link between yoga and spine health. One study published in the journal *Pain* found that people who attended a weekly yoga class and practiced at home reported 70 percent less lower-back pain after 3 months. What's more, 88 percent of them either used less pain medication or stopped taking it altogether. (Only 35 percent of a yoga-deprived control group did.) How does yoga help? The poses help correct imbalances in the musculoskeletal system affecting spinal alignment and posture. Practicing this routine twice a week will increase your awareness of how you move your body, helping you learn to maintain a healthy posture.

the **ROUTINE**

Try the following sequence, staying in each pose for 5 deep inhales and exhales, unless otherwise noted.

Standing Forward Bend, Elbow Hold
p. 31

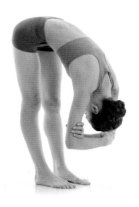

Squat Twist
p. 35

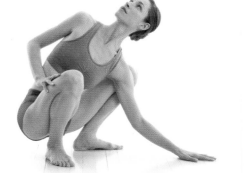

Back Lengthener
with Easy Twist
p. 32

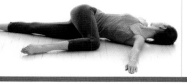

Squat Hang
p. 35

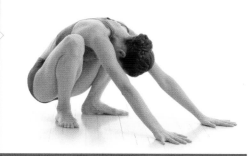

Spine Twist
p. 125

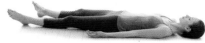

Corpse
p. 126

After resting in corpse for 5 breaths, carefully roll your body to the right side. Rest here for a few breaths and gently come up to sit.

Go back to the beginning and repeat the entire sequence on the other side.

TAKE IT FROM
Tara

BABY YOUR BACK

Not all back pain is equal. Listen to your body and know your limitations. Pushing and forcing yourself into a position won't do you any good and often can hurt you. Use your breath to guide you: Move a little bit each time you take a breath, rather than forcing yourself all at once into any position. Do only what you can do easily and what feels right for your body. If you take it easy and give yourself time, you'll find your way to what your body needs.

Carpal Tunnel Syndrome

The carpal tunnel is a narrow passageway located on the palm side of your wrist. Its job is to protect an important nerve that leads to your hand and the nine tendons that bend your fingers.

Whether it's for work, staying connected to friends, reading the news, or having fun, you probably spend more hours than you think tapping some kind of keyboard. All that typing and clicking can place excessive pressure on the nerve, and over time that can result in numbness, pain, and hand weakness. This constellation of symptoms is known as carpal tunnel syndrome (CTS).

If you've ever had carpal tunnel problems, you know they suck. That's why I'm happy to tell you that yoga can work wonders for your wrists. In a study at the University of Pennsylvania, researchers divided a group of patients with CTS into two groups. Twice a week for 8 weeks, one group followed a program of relaxation techniques and yoga postures. Patients in the other group received wrist splints. After the study period, the yoga group experienced a major improvement in grip strength and significant pain reduction. The patients in the control group did not.

the **ROUTINE**

Do this sequence three times a week to strengthen your wrists and relieve pain.

Palm Raise
p. 42

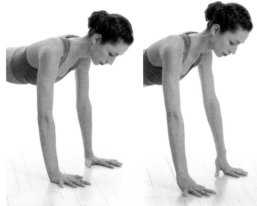

With a slow, continuous motion, raise and lower your palms 10 times. Repeat 10 times with your fingers pointing outward and 10 times pointing inward.

Standing Hand Step
p. 33

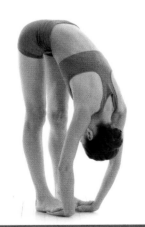

Hold for 5 long, deep inhales and exhales.

Fists Facing

p. 44

Hold the straightest position you can with tight fists for 3 long, deep inhales and exhales. Repeat this 3 times.

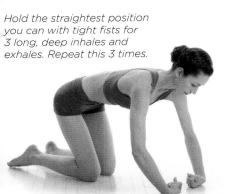

Wrist Release

p. 45

Hold for 3 long, deep inhales and exhales. Slowly release and switch sides.

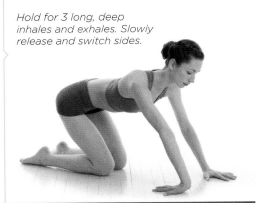

Standing Palm Press

p. 29

Hold for 5 long, deep inhales and exhales.

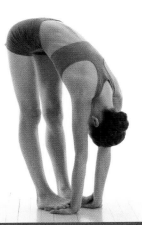

Digestive Problems

For anyone who's ever had to run to the bathroom before a stressful presentation or meeting, I have good news: A regular yoga practice can ease your belly woes.

As I've mentioned in previous sections, stress triggers the part of your nervous system that's responsible for the fight-or-flight response, which can wreak havoc on your stomach. Fortunately yoga, breathing, and meditation activate the part of your nervous system responsible for relaxation, which helps counteract stress reactions.

One study in India looked at the effect of yoga versus conventional medication in patients with a form of irritable bowel syndrome characterized by bouts of diarrhea. Luckily for the subjects in this study, both the yoga and the medication helped. But the patients who had the good fortune to be assigned to the yoga group enjoyed additional benefits: Researchers documented changes in the balance of their nervous systems in favor of the area responsible for relaxation.

Try the following routine twice a week to maintain overall digestive health. It's important to listen to your body to get the most out of your practice, and also to avoid further imbalance and injury. If a pose doesn't feel right for your body at the time, skip it.

the
ROUTINE

Hold each pose for 20 deep inhales and exhales.

Child's Pose Twist
p. 93

Do to one side, then the other.

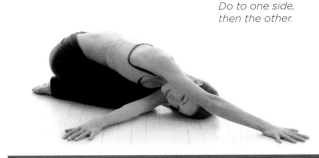

Shoulder Stand
p. 114

Legs up the Wall
p. 114

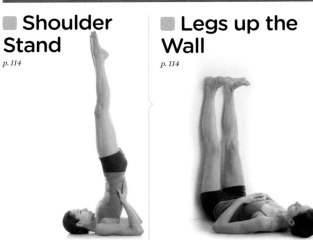

Sit on Heels
p. 93

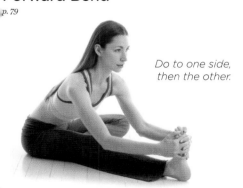

Plow
p. 112

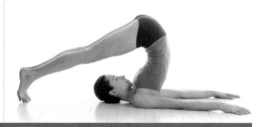

Seated Single-Leg Forward Bend
p. 79

Do to one side, then the other.

Seated Forward Bend, Bent Knees
p. 76

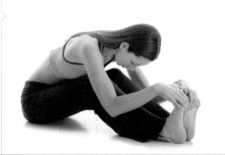

Hangovers

I'm going to give it to you straight: There's not a drop of research to back up the effect of yoga on a nasty hangover (though it has been proven to help the symptoms; see "Headaches" on page 238 and "Vertigo" on page 248). But who cares when you just want the room to stop spinning and your head to stop hurting, right?

You may not feel like moving from your bed, but if you can crawl to your yoga mat, there are a few easy moves that will get you on the road to recovery. They may even have you back to your usual self in less time than it takes for the aspirin to kick in.

the **ROUTINE**

Do what you can to make it over to your yoga mat. If that just isn't going to happen this morning, you can try most of these poses from your bed. Wait until you can make it to your mat for the headstand, though.

Try the following sequence, staying in each pose for 10 deep inhales and exhales, unless otherwise noted.

◼ Hero
p. 86

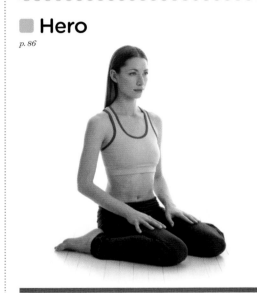

◼ Easy Hero Twist
p. 87

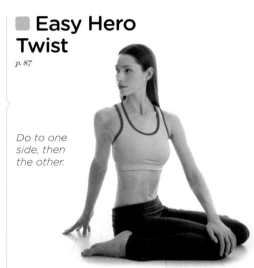

Do to one side, then the other.

◼ Child's Pose
p. 92

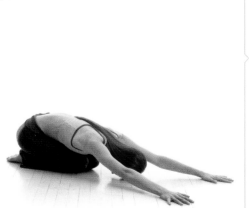

◼ Seated Spine Twist
p. 81

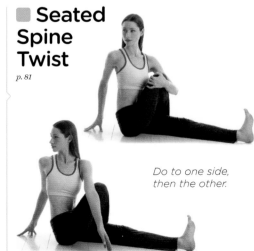

Do to one side, then the other.

Headstand Prep, Feet Walked In
p. 104

Headstand Prep, Both Heels to Hips
p. 105

Headstand
p. 106

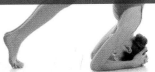

Feel free to skip the headstand sequence if you are new to headstand. If you want to give it a try, practice each stage until you feel comfortable in it, then move on to the next stage.

Seated Forward Bend
p. 74

Supported Corpse with Blocks
p. 127

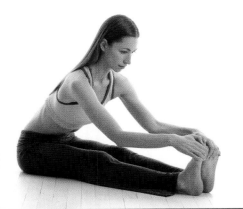
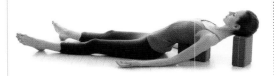

HEADSTAND HELP

If you have never done a headstand, it's best not to attempt your first on a morning after you partied a little too hard. Headstands require concentration and alertness. You can always try when you're feeling better. Even if you are a headstand pro, make sure to take your time, pay attention, and ease into it slowly. If you do make it into the pose, the detoxifying and revitalizing effects are fantastic. Headstand stimulates and rejuvenates the endocrine, circulatory, lymphatic, nervous, and respiratory systems. Headstands also calm the mind.

Headaches

Headaches can be caused by stress, anxiety, dehydration, or exhaustion. They can pop up out of nowhere or creep their way in gradually.

There's a whole pharmaceutical-based industry devoted to easing headache symptoms, but science also backs yoga as a less invasive alternative. Researchers in India compared the outcomes of treating headache patients with nonsteroidal anti-inflammatories (such as ibuprofen), Botox injections (yes, this wrinkle smoother is approved for headache relief), and yoga. The patients treated with yoga reported less pain than the patients treated with the other methods. Step away from the lethal bacteria, people!

In another study, researchers randomly assigned migraine sufferers to 3 months of either a yoga intervention or self-care. Guess who reported significantly reduced migraine frequency and pain? Yep, the om team.

When you feel the pressures of the day weighing you down, take the time to reduce anxiety levels and open up some space in your brain. Try this routine three times a week while you're sitting at your desk, either at work or at home. If your job is physical, find a quiet place to sit for a few minutes.

the ROUTINE

Hold each pose for 5 deep inhales and exhales.

THREE WISE MONKEYS

◻ Eye Soother
p. 84

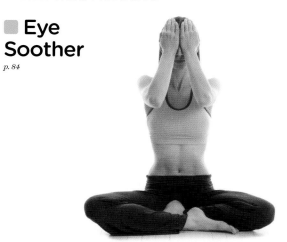

◻ Alternate Nostril Breathing
p. 15

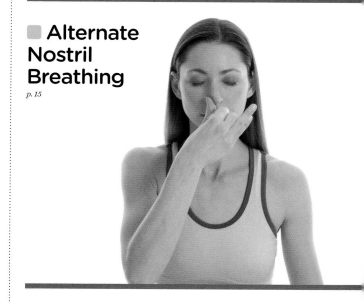

ACCORDING TO THE ancient Three Wise Monkeys maxim, to be anxiety free is to be free of evil happening to us, or in yoga philosophy, evil that we inflict upon ourselves. The ancient yogis believed suffering is a choice. We can choose to be happy and free from our circumstances or attached to them. When we let go of them, we have an inner calm, no matter what is happening in our lives. Only with practice are we free from the roller coaster of emotions.

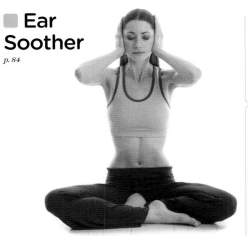

Ear Soother
p. 84

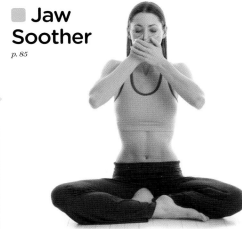

Jaw Soother
p. 85

Temple Massage

Stay in your seated position and press your index and middle fingers of both hands gently on your forehead between your eyebrows. Hold here for a few breaths. Press gently upward on your forehead and then slide your fingers down toward your temples. Press in and up on your temples and hold here for 3 long, deep breaths. Repeat 3 times.

WATER WORKS

Headaches are often related to dehydration. You could reach for some pills as a quick fix, but keeping hydrated might be a better option. In one study, Dutch researchers asked a group of headache sufferers to increase their water intake over a period of 12 weeks. The result? Headache duration and intensity decreased. The subjects increased the amount they drank by 1.5 liters a day. (That's a little more than six 8-ounce glasses.) Keep a glass or bottle with you while you're working. It's easy to get dehydrated, whether you're staring at the computer screen for hours on end or running around doing errands.

Heart Disease

Heart disease is the number one killer of women over 25 in this country. It kills more women than all cancers combined. That's scary. Fortunately, practicing yoga can help you sidestep the consequences of this devastating disease. Numerous studies have linked yoga to reducing body weight (see chapter 4) and lowering blood pressure and cholesterol, all major contributors to heart disease.

Heart rate variability, a sign of a healthy heart, also has been shown to be greater in yoga practitioners than in nonpractitioners, according to a 2009 study in the *International Journal of Medical Engineering and Informatics*.

Using the breath to strengthen the body and release tension provides you with an ample flow of oxygen and promotes a healthy heart. And according to research from Yale University School of Medicine, people who practice yoga and meditation at least three times a week lower their blood pressure, their pulse, and their risk of heart disease. To protect your ticker, practice this sequence twice a week.

the **ROUTINE**

Try the following sequence, staying in each pose for 10 deep inhales and exhales, unless otherwise noted.

■ **Chair**
p. 61
with Breath of Fire
p. 15

Breath of fire will get you warm and get your heart pumping, and holding a chair pose will get the muscles in your whole body involved.

In your chair pose, start to increase your rate of even inhales and exhales until you are rapidly pumping air in and out of your body. Hold the breath pattern for 30 seconds. Return to standing. Repeat 3 times. If 30 seconds feels like a long time, start with shorter periods and work from there.

■ **Seated Meditation,**
Arms in V
p. 70

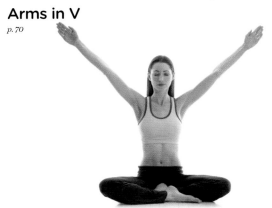

Low Lunge
p. 46

Do to one side, then the other.

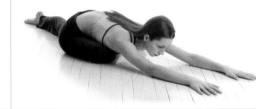

Pigeon
p. 90

Do to one side, then the other.

Seated Meditation
p. 69

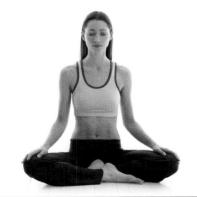

Infertility

Pregnancy can be a surprise, the outcome of precise planning, or the result of a long and frustrating process. So many factors contribute to infertility, and not everything can be solved by logical means. There's not a ton of research that links yoga directly to boundless fertility. But because of yoga's proven ability to lower stress and anxiety levels, Herbert Benson, the Harvard doctor famous for identifying the relaxation response, has included yoga for years in his Mind-Body Program for Health and Fertility at Massachusetts General Hospital in Boston. And when researchers studied a group of women who had been trying »

the ROUTINE

Try the following sequence, staying in each pose for 15 deep inhales and exhales.

☐ Low Lunge
p. 46

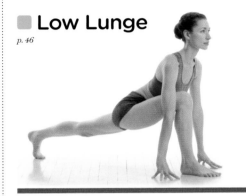

☐ Low Lunge, Back Knee Down, Hip Release (Lizard)
p. 49

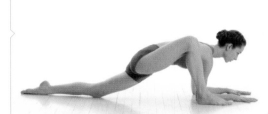

☐ Down Dog
p. 36

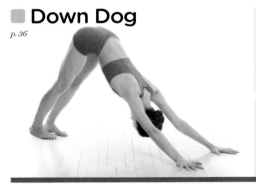

☐ Down Dog Split
p. 38

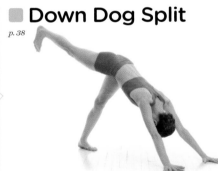

☐ Standing Forward Bend,
Neck Release
p. 31

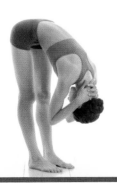

☐ Squat
p. 34

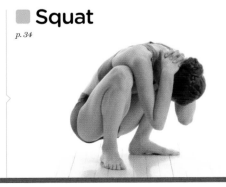

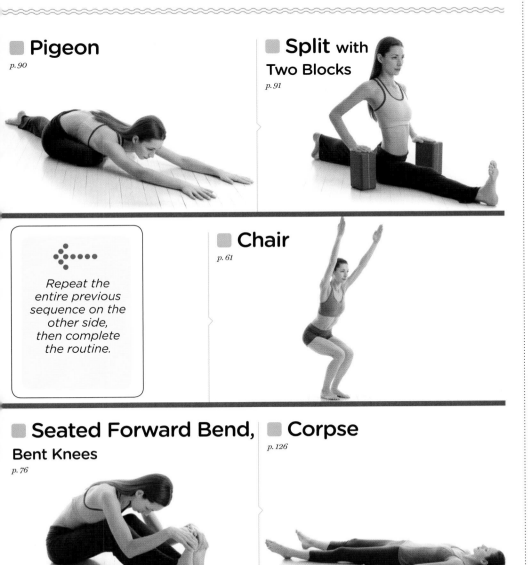

Pigeon
p. 90

Split with Two Blocks
p. 91

Repeat the entire previous sequence on the other side, then complete the routine.

Chair
p. 61

Seated Forward Bend, Bent Knees
p. 76

Corpse
p. 126

» to conceive for 1 to 2 years and were enrolled in a program similar to Benson's, they found something pretty hopeful: 55 percent became pregnant. Of those pregnancies, nearly half occurred without the help of any baby-making technology, such as in vitro fertilization. Yoga certainly wasn't the only thing at work here (guided imagery, deep breathing, and group therapy are also part of the program), but researchers attribute the success in part to yoga's stress-busting power.

If you're trying to make a baby, give your body the best possible chance by practicing this routine 2 or 3 times a week.

Jet Lag

When you have a bad case of sluggishness after a long flight, yoga might just help you adjust. Scientists at Northwestern University and the University of California at San Francisco biopsied muscle samples from people who had performed resistance exercise and found changes in the muscle proteins that regulate circadian rhythms. Their conclusion? Resistance training (like the challenging body-weight-bearing lunges in this routine) may help your body adjust to time zone changes.

Head for your mat as soon as you reach your destination and try these poses to reset your body and mind.

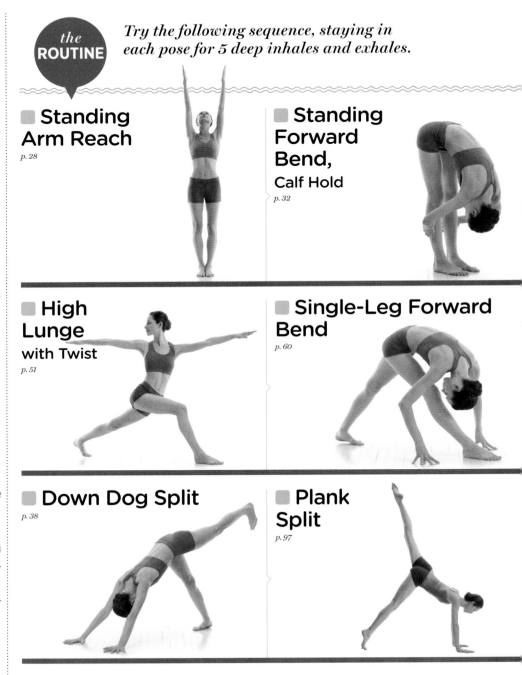

the ROUTINE

Try the following sequence, staying in each pose for 5 deep inhales and exhales.

Standing Arm Reach
p. 28

Standing Forward Bend, Calf Hold
p. 32

High Lunge with Twist
p. 51

Single-Leg Forward Bend
p. 60

Down Dog Split
p. 38

Plank Split
p. 97

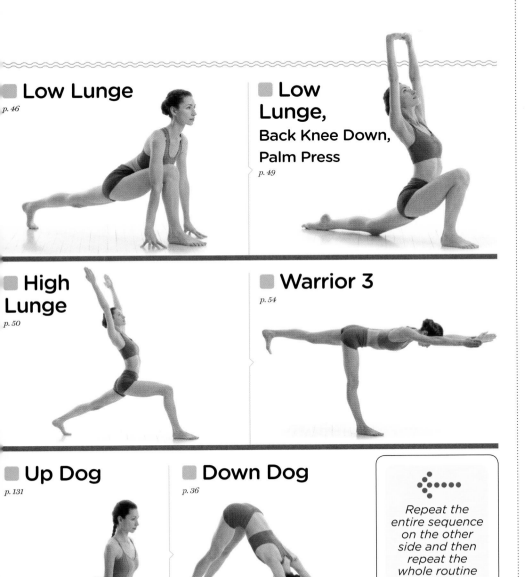

Low Lunge
p. 46

Low Lunge,
**Back Knee Down,
Palm Press**
p. 49

High Lunge
p. 50

Warrior 3
p. 54

Up Dog
p. 131

Down Dog
p. 36

Repeat the entire sequence on the other side and then repeat the whole routine (left and right sides) 3 more times.

Pregnancy

People often ask me if it's safe to practice yoga while they're pregnant. Use common sense: Check with your doctor before trying anything new, and don't do anything you're not completely comfortable with. That said, it's worth knowing that research has shown that practicing yoga during pregnancy is not only safe, but also beneficial to the baby and mother. A study published in the *Journal of Alternative and Complementary Therapy* divided 335 pregnant women into two groups. One group practiced yoga regularly; the other walked 30 minutes twice a day. The women in the yoga group had fewer low-birth-weight babies than the walkers did, as well as less preterm labor, fewer complications, and no increased risk of complications.

Practicing breathing and listening to your body and mind can also ease anxiety, tension, and fears that go along with pregnancy. When you feel pain or become afraid—which can happen when you're trying to push out a baby the size of a KitchenAid mixer—your body produces extra adrenaline (the fight-or-flight hormone). When that hormone starts pumping, it slows down your body's other functions—in this case, the production of the hormone that causes contractions. That makes for a long, »

the ROUTINE

Try the following sequence, staying in each pose for 5 deep inhales and exhales, unless otherwise noted.

◼ Chair Meditation

Sit up tall on a chair. (A chair with a back is a little more restorative.) Make sure both feet are flat on the floor and your spine is lengthening up tall. Relax your shoulders away from your ears. Gently place your hands on your lap, close your eyes, and follow your breath. Breathe here for a few minutes. Lift a little weight out of your body with each inhale, and relax a little more with each exhale. Press down on the chair with your hands and gently stand up.

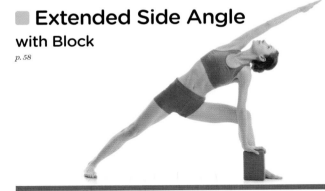

◼ Extended Side Angle
with Block
p. 58

◼ Seated Shin Hug
p. 80

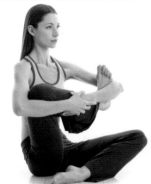

Hug one shin, then the other.

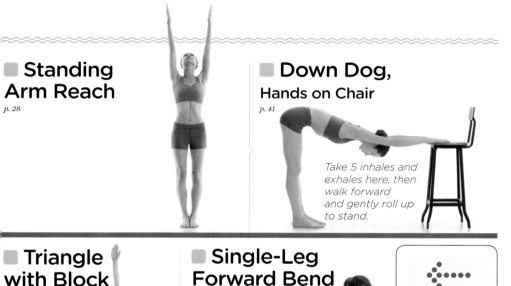

▪ Standing Arm Reach
p. 28

▪ Down Dog,
Hands on Chair
p. 41

Take 5 inhales and exhales here, then walk forward and gently roll up to stand.

▪ Triangle with Block
p. 57

▪ Single-Leg Forward Bend
with Blocks
p. 59

Repeat the whole sequence on the other side before finishing with the shin hug.

TAKE IT FROM

Tara

YOGA
WITH A
BUMP

Most experts in prenatal yoga advise that if you have never practiced yoga and want to start while pregnant, to practice prenatal yoga only. If you've maintained a regular yoga practice before becoming pregnant, experts say it's safe to continue with that.

Practice during the first trimester should be very gentle, because the fetus is still implanting. By the second trimester, most women can continue with regular practice. By the third trimester, experts suggest using a wall or chair to help with balance. Some prenatal teachers advise against lying on your back during the third trimester. Others say it's okay for short periods of time.

» uncomfortable labor. But yoga has been shown to make pregnancy and labor less taxing: A 2009 study at the University of Minnesota's School of Nursing found that practicing yoga reduced pain and decreased stress levels in pregnant women. And a 2008 study published in the journal *Complementary Therapies in Clinical Practice* found that patients who practiced yoga reported lower levels of pain during delivery and had shorter total delivery times. To minimize discomfort during pregnancy and prep your body for a more manageable delivery, try this routine twice a week when you've got a bun in the oven.

Vertigo

Vertigo is one of the most common health problems in adults. According to the National Institutes of Health, about 40 percent of people in the United States experience it, and it's more common in women. If you have vertigo, the feeling of spinning and motion sickness can be overwhelming and is often triggered by the slightest movement. Some causes of vertigo are poor circulation, infections, allergies, and neurological diseases. While scientists haven't specifically studied the effect of yoga on vertigo, a number of studies have looked at how yoga benefits chemotherapy patients: One side effect of chemo »

the **ROUTINE**

Try the following sequence, staying in each pose for 10 deep inhales and exhales.

■ Squat
p. 34

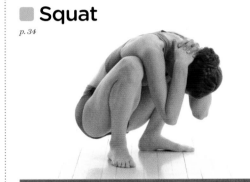

■ Standing Forward Bend,
Elbow Hold
p. 31

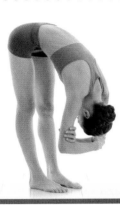

■ Sit on Heels
p. 93

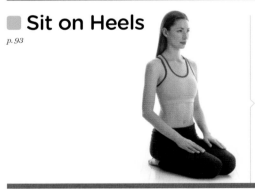

■ Headstand Prep,
Feet Walked In
p. 104

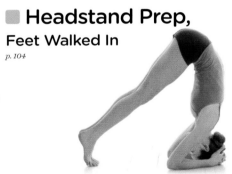

■ Plow
p. 112

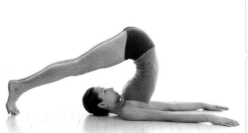

■ Corpse
p. 126

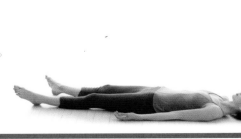

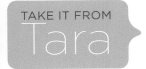
LET THE FEELING PASS

Take it easy. If you become dizzy in yoga class, don't push through a pose. It's fine to sit up on your heels, breathe and allow the sensation to pass. Practicing this kind of patience with yourself, while listening to your body, is just as valuable as any other part of yoga.

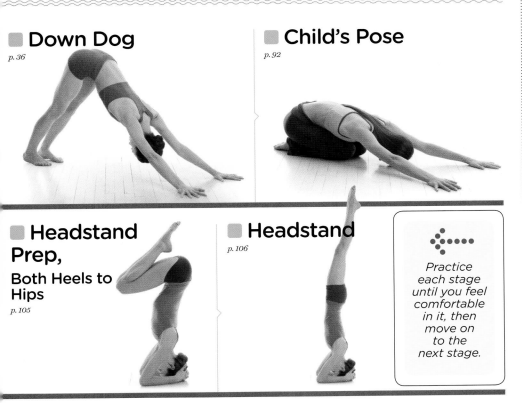

Down Dog
p. 36

Child's Pose
p. 92

Headstand Prep,
Both Heels to Hips
p. 105

Headstand
p. 106

Practice each stage until you feel comfortable in it, then move on to the next stage.

» is debilitating nausea, which is similar to what people with vertigo experience. In a 2007 study published in the *European Journal of Cancer Care*, researchers randomly assigned cancer patients to receive either a yoga intervention or psychological therapy during the course of their chemo. At the end of the trial, the yoga group had reduced nausea frequency and intensity compared with the therapy patients.

Yoga can ease vertigo by building focus and concentration, reducing anxiety, and stimulating the nervous system. This routine is designed to reduce anxiety by helping the body and mind adjust to being upside down. Try this sequence three times a week.

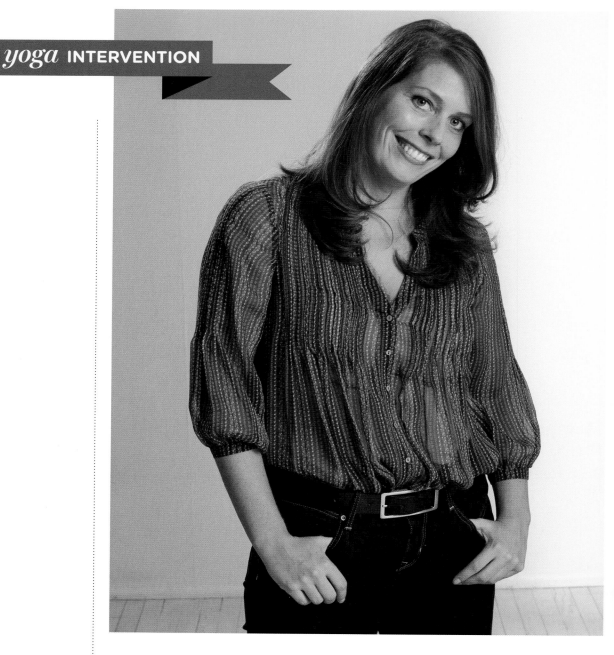

Lindsay Mannering

THE ISSUE: **VERTIGO**

"Go beyond your comfort zone. Each time you do, your comfort zone gets bigger and bigger. Pretty soon, you'll be doing things you never thought you could do."

Lindsay has had vertigo since she played sports in grade school. "I'd get dizzy and have to sit down to stop the spinning," says the 28-year-old sales manager.

"Now that I'm an adult, I can't just sit down any time it strikes." And it strikes unpredictably. The nausea and dizziness can start during a meeting, in an elevator, or at lunch with a friend. It's completely random. Sometimes a few days go by without an episode, and sometimes it happens more frequently. "It makes getting things done really hard," she says.

After her doctor couldn't pinpoint a medical reason for her spinning spells, Lindsay's sister, a physical therapist, recommended she try yoga. "At first, I got dizzy any time I bent over in down dog," Lindsay says. "I pretty much couldn't stand it any time my head was lower than my heart." But after several weeks, her tolerance improved, and she learned to work with her body instead of fighting it. "It's become easier to let the symptoms come and go," she says. "Pushing past my comfort zone helped me realize that I'd be OK even if I felt a little dizzy."

It's still a challenge, but bending over on the mat has started feeling good. "The more I practice yoga, the less it makes me spin!" she says. And Lindsay feels better off the mat, too.

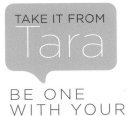

TAKE IT FROM
Tara

BE ONE WITH YOUR BODY

We spend a lot of our lives working against our bodies, gathering stress that leads to health problems. Yoga helps you work with your body so you can set aside stress and stay healthy.

take it
to the
next level

Everything you need to live yoga

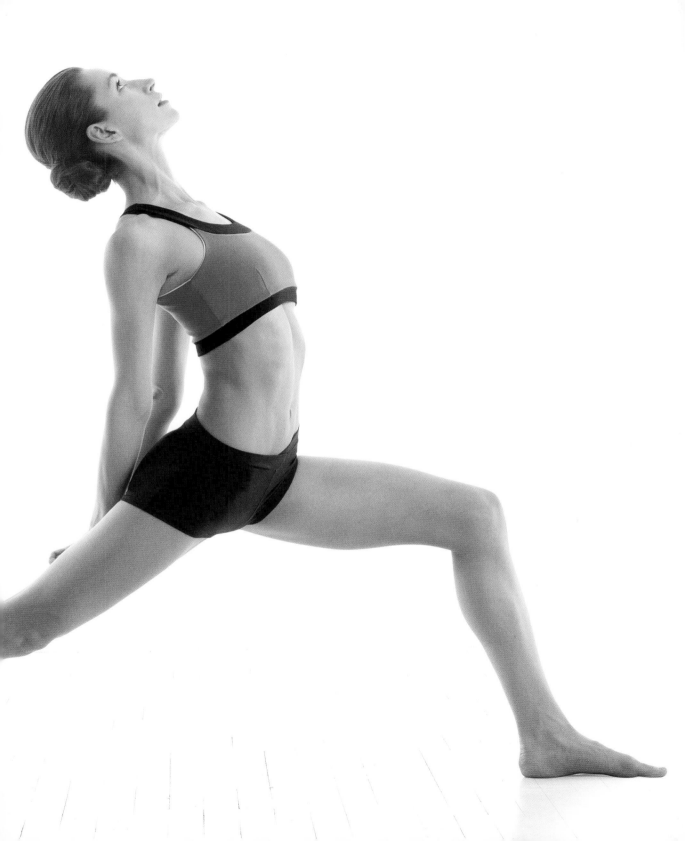

After reading this book and noticing the difference just 15 minutes of yoga a day can make, you may find yourself wanting more. You may suddenly notice the racks of yoga outfits at Target, or the social aspect of a class might lure you to a studio, or you may want the personal attention of a real live teacher to help you get the most from your practice.

Consider this final chapter your yoga cheat sheet for must-have equipment, how to find a class or teacher, what kind of yoga is right for you, and how to achieve the yoga mindset that will set you on the right track toward reaching all your goals.

Yoga Gear

You'll definitely need some comfortable clothes to practice yoga in, but before you buy up all the latest yoga fashions, put your paycheck in the bank and go shopping in your closet. Regular gym clothes like a sports bra, tank top, pants, and shorts work fine. Other options are old T-shirts and sweatpants. You want to be comfortable and able to move. Try to avoid anything too bulky that might fall over your head when you go upside down. If you start practicing yoga at home, pajama bottoms and a bra top are a good, comfy option. I prefer loose cotton drawstring pants and a tank top. That's pretty much my uniform.

If you decide eventually that your worn-in college sweats and old boyfriend's tee are hindering your progress, here are a few ideas.

Most chain stores like Target, Walmart, and Dick's carry yoga-specific apparel. Try on a few options to see what works for you. Consider making eco-friendly choices when you shop for yoga duds. The more yoga you practice, the more you will be concerned about how you live and your affect on the world. There's something about all that inward focus and deep breathing that breeds compassion for ourselves, others, and the planet. A growing number of brands and stores offer planet-friendly yoga duds, including brands like Gaiam, Blue Canoe, and Alternative Apparel, all of which are available online.

You'll be able to incorporate many of the routines in this book so seamlessly into your life that you might not feel the need for a yoga mat. That said, it's nice to have one lying around the house somewhere, ready for spontaneous practice. I keep one rolled out on my living room floor for inspiration. If it's right there staring back at me, I practice much more often than if it was stored in the corner somewhere.

Your mat choice can play a big part in your overall reaction to yoga. A mat made of plastic and other synthetic materials can be slippery and provide an uncomfortable experience right from your first down dog. Mats made of rubber or other eco-friendly materials are your best bet, because they aren't slippery and are thick enough to provide cushioning. Many yoga teachers and practitioners suggest Manduka and Jade mats. Pick your favorite color to inspire you to spend more time on it.

A lot of the routines in this book call for blocks, which can help support you and ease you into certain poses. Occasionally I also suggest using a rolled-up towel or blanket for support. You usually can purchase straps or blocks wherever yoga gear is sold.

If you decide to take a class, studios should have everything you need. Some teachers incorporate straps and blankets into practice. You can save in this department by bringing a towel or blanket that you already have at home. It's worth knowing that while many studios provide mats, some charge an extra fee for them, and studio mats can sometimes be breeding grounds for germs. One more reason to consider investing in your own.

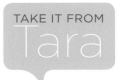

TAKE IT FROM
Tara

GOOD MORNING ALERT!

Beware. Practicing yoga can lead to happiness. The more you incorporate yoga routines into your day, the better you'll feel. All the deep breathing and down dogs put you back in touch with your creativity and peel away the layers of stress. Prepare to feel great.

How to Find a Class

There are so many different teachers and styles of yoga now that it can be hard to decide which is best for you without test-driving a bunch. Certification requirements run the gamut from a weekend course to multiple years. Most teachers list in their bios where they studied, with whom, for how long, and what certificates they hold. Many teachers are listed with an association called the Yoga Alliance. It's tricky, though, because all schools of yoga are different, and even if someone has many years of training, you still may not like their style. It's also worth noting, especially if you hope yoga will help resolve a health problem, that most yoga teachers aren't medical professionals. If you need a health diagnosis, turn to a medical professional.

You might need to studio-hop for a couple of months until you find a style, studio, and teacher that you vibe with. It may be as simple as finding the studio closest to your job that has class at a time that works for you. Or you may find yourself schlepping across town to a class with a teacher you can't get enough of. Here are my insider tips for finding instruction you'll want to stick with.

GOOGLE IT UP. There are whole studios dedicated to pre- and postnatal, meditation, athletic, or gentle yoga, and more. Some emphasize the spiritual aspects of yoga more than others. Look for that information on the studio or teacher's website. Google the studio and your teacher's name for testimonials, mentions in blogs, and reviews on Web sites.

ASK AROUND. Some teachers lead the class in chanting. Some emphasize pose perfection. Some pick favorite students. One of the best ways to get details on a teacher's style is through word of mouth. Ask friends and people who have similar interests and goals to yours, and you'll probably get sent in the right direction. Bottom line: Your yoga teacher should be kind, knowledge-able, and excited to teach yoga.

LOOK NEXT DOOR. Just for the sake of convenience, check out the nearest yoga studio to your home or job. Wouldn't it be nice to be able to roll out your mat just a few blocks away from where you are right now?

CONSIDER YOUR SCHEDULE. Most yoga classes are between an hour and an hour and a half in length. Times are usually listed on studios' websites. Think about how much time you have to devote to yoga, since travel time can add up.

LOOK FOR YOGA IN UNEX-PECTED PLACES. Although yoga studios are almost as prevalent as Starbucks in major cities, they are still just trickling into suburbs and smaller towns. Check your local gym and other community spaces for classes. The small town where I grew up (Morris, Illinois) offers yoga classes at the local hospital and library. Still no yoga? iTunes has some useful video and audio classes, which are a great way to bring your favorite big-name teacher right to your living room. DVDs are also a great tool when you find a teacher you really like. (And of course, this book is packed with a ton of routines and tips!)

First Yoga Class Ever? A Few Tips . . .

Once you have a class all picked out, here's how to have the best experience possible.

■ **CHECK FOR REQUIREMENTS.** The studio may ask you to fill out a first-timer form and waiver before class, or recommend that you take a certain class if you are brand new to yoga. Check the studio website for this information, and call if you have further questions.

■ **SAVE YOUR BIG MEAL FOR AFTER.** It's better to practice yoga when your stomach isn't full. A stuffed belly can make all that twisting and deep breathing uncomfortable and limit your potential. If you are starving and it's close to class time, grab something small and easy to digest, like a piece of fruit that will hold you over.

■ **DRINK WATER.** You should be drinking water whether you're headed to yoga class or not, and it's a good idea to hydrate before and after your class to keep your system running smoothly. For most styles of yoga, drinking about 8 ounces before class and about 8 ounces after should keep you hydrated. Some studios suggest that you don't drink water during the class so you can focus all your attention on the practice. If you're well hydrated before the class, you should be fine waiting to drink water until after. The one exception: Bikram yoga. Because these classes take place in rooms where the thermostats are set at a minimum of 105°F, you'll sweat a lot more than in a regular class. If you're into Bikram, the Yoga Research and Education Center suggests drinking at least the minimum recommended daily 64 ounces of water, plus 16 ounces before and at least 20 ounces during class.

■ **SHOW UP A LITTLE EARLY.** Ten to 15 minutes leaves plenty of time to sign in and get a good spot.

■ **SAY HI TO THE TEACHER.** Let him or her know it's your first class at the studio or first time practicing yoga, and whether you have any specific limitations or injuries.

■ **TAKE IT EASY.** Don't push or fling yourself into the poses. Try to keep your breathing long and deep. If your breathing becomes short and fast, ease up to where you can bring it back to long and deep. Long, deep breathing helps you move calmly and attentively through challenging and unchallenging poses alike, and will give you the most benefits from the poses. Deep breathing helps your body open up and your mind rest. It takes practice. It may take a lot of time to be able to master the poses you want, but remember that once you do, there will always be something else to master. Start from where you are. Where you are is perfect.

What's Your Yoga Personality?

Check out this chart to match your personality and preferences with the right yoga style for you. You can always challenge yourself more or take a rest during class to adjust to what you can handle physically. Remember that spirituality is what you make of it. Certain styles deliberately lead you to it; others let you find your own way to whatever you want. Some styles of yoga begin with a chant or an opening collective om, some include chanting throughout the class, and some skip it completely.

YOGA STYLE	CHARACTERISTICS	SWEAT METER	CHANT METER	GOOD WHEN . . .
Ananda	Gentle yoga poses with focus on meditation rather than athleticism.	Low	High: Lots of chanting at the beginning and end of class.	You want a gentle physical practice that focuses on meditation.
Anusara	Poses are taught with a strong alignment focus coupled with playful themes.	Low	High: Lengthy opening invocation and closing om.	You like a tight-knit yoga community that is known for its playful approach.
Ashtanga	Athletic and challenging poses. Fast-paced movement. Often jumping forward and back.	High	High: Opening and closing lengthy chant.	You want a strong physical and spiritual practice.
Bikram	26-posture series. Same every class. Done in a 105°F room.	High	Low: No chanting.	Sweating buckets is a requirement, and you don't mind heat.
Iyengar	Poses are taught with a strong focus on alignment. Class works on perfecting one pose at a time.	Medium	Medium: Depends on the teacher.	You want to focus on alignment and the technical aspects of the poses.
Kundalini	Primarily seated positions coupled with vigorous breathing techniques.	Medium	High: Lots of chanting at the beginning and end of class.	You're interested in developing a strong meditative practice.
Vinyasa	Athletic poses. Covers a wide range of levels of difficulty, depending on the teacher.	Medium to high	Medium: An opening and closing om is common but is sometimes left out. Depends on the teacher.	You want a workout and like to move with your breath, often to music.

Index

Boldface page references indicate photographs. <u>Underscored</u> references indicate boxed text.